Ageing slowly, Living longer

Perceptions and Visions for Longevity

Vinod Nikhra

Published by
InnoSpan
Spandan Innovative

Published by
InnoSpan
(Spandan Innovative)

In association with
Kindle Direct Publishing - KDP

ISBN: 9798684775871

Copyright © Vinod Nikhra 2022

Ageing slowly, Living longer
Perceptions and Visions for Longevity
Dr Vinod Nikhra M.D.

.

Vinod Nikhra

Ageing slowly, Living longer

Perceptions and Visions for Longevity

InnoSpan

Books by the Author

COVID-19: Perspective, Patterns and
Evolving strategies (eBook)

Living with COVID-19: The Nemesis, the Hubris
and the Elpis (eBook)

COVID-19 and Long Covid: Organ damage and
Dysfunctions, and Implications for Clinical Course
(eBook)

Date with the Pandemic: Perspective, Disease
and Aftermath

Doctor, doctor:
Intimate stories from doctors' lives
(Book one)

Doctor's den:
Intimate stories from doctors' lives
(Book Two)

Doctors' world:
Intimate stories from doctors' lives
(Book Three)

Something Like Love – Intimate stories
(Fiction)

The Anti-obesity Guide
(Non-fiction)

*****

Wonderful advances in the field of medical science make possible to slow down ageing process and live a long and healthy life. The author has, to share with you, the facts and visions more eloquent than imaginations and amazing thoughts amounting to reality-pregnant-early-morning dreams.

It may seem, but the work is not a fiction. Neither it is a bundle of concocted myths. Based on current state of scientific knowledge and gerontological research, the book aims to provide answers to mystery of ageing and disease processes. Simultaneously, it is designed to help to preserve health and fitness.

Therefore, you are requested to read on. After all, the theme, ageing slowly and living longer, is of a prime interest to all of us.

*****

Dr Vinod Nikhra M.D. is the Convenor of Longevity Research Group. He is a physician and trained in internal medicine, clinical cardiology, nephrology, endocrinology and health management. He has done Clinical Observer-ship in internal medicine at East Alabama Medical Center, Opelika, U.S.A. He has special interest in cardiology, diabetology, neurology, gerontology and geriatrics, rheumatology, haematology, and nano-biotechnology. He is associated as Overseas Fellow with Royal society of Medicine, London, as Fellow with International Medical Sciences Academy, and as Member with Cardiological Society of India, Indian College of Interventional Cardiology, Association of Physicians of India, Indian Society of Nephrology, Indian Society of Haemodialysis, Asian Pacific Society of Nephrology, National Kidney Foundation USA, Alumni Association of Department of Nephrology, IMS Banaras Hindu University; Indian Society of Rheumatology, Indian Society of Haematology and Indian Medical Association; apart from various regional medical societies. He is the President of Association for Health in Middle Aged (AHIMA). Above all, he loves writing and over the years he has written widely acclaimed fiction and non-fiction books. He has been Founder-editor of "MADHYA: the midage", Journal of AHIMA.

He lives with his wife Rashmi, son Vibhor, daughter-in-law Archana and daughter Vindhya, and dog Yuki, in New Delhi, India.

*****

Dedicated to

Beloved Nannaji,

Late Shri Ram Nath Nikhra

my mentor and granduncle, and

a prolific writer

*****

Introduction
Welcome to the World of Longevity

A DISEASE OF MODERN TIMES

The world today is fast progressing, and we live in the unprecedented times. There is a boom of advances in every field, from the art to the science and technology. This includes health science, too. There are fascinating stories of human endeavour. The wonderful advances in the field of medical science make it possible to cure acute disorders and, thus, avoiding untimely demise. The chronic diseases like obesity, diabetes, high blood pressure, heart disease, etc. can be efficiently managed leading to virtual freedom from their complications. There is, in general, an appreciable increase in life expectancy and lifespan.

The modern day, high-tech interventions and revolutionized medicine enable us to maintain a good level of function well into the later years. Albeit we should not forget that one is responsible for one's own health. Here lies the importance of self-help, lifestyle choices and role of health guidance (Fig 1).

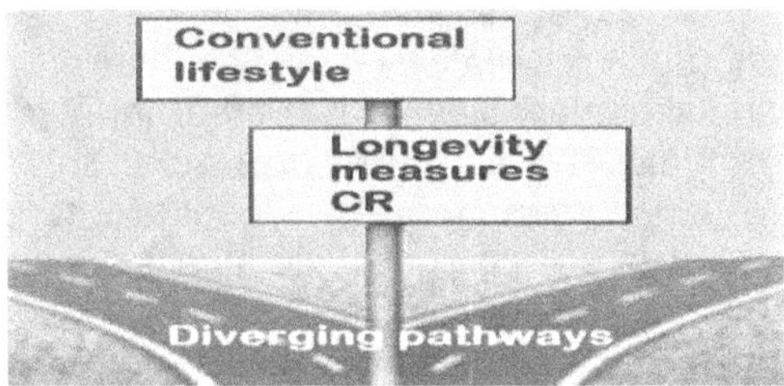

Figure 1: Lifestyle choices for healthy longevity

Increasingly doctors are encouraging people to become active participants in managing their own health by following a healthy lifestyle and sticking to optimal health behaviours. Today, the behavioral approaches are being successfully applied to disabling conditions such as obesity, diabetes mellitus, high blood pressure, heart disease, cognitive disorders and disabling conditions like urinary incontinence. Because lifestyle is so critical to health, more time should be devoted to lifestyle interventions which, should be tailored to requirements of an ageing individual and group.

There are certain important emerging issues in the modern health scenario. A good number of people are surviving in their sixties and seventies and entering into the post-retirement phase of life. With better medical care and public health efforts, there is an increased average life expectancy in general and improved survival rates in particular. There are two different views on the trend: a pessimistic view emphasizing an increased burden on healthcare due to age-related illnesses and disability; and an optimistic view regarding postponement of chronic illness and disability during the later years due to improved lifestyles and better healthcare. The population and clinical studies, too, reveal declining disease and disability rates and support the optimistic view.

The clinical, behavioural, and social risk factors are important. The co-morbidities, which are the hallmark of ageing, make the disease management especially challenging during the later years. The double burden of obesity and sedentary lifestyle is a predictor of increased incidence of diabetes and heart disease. In this context, there are widespread benefits attributable to physical activity, but a large number of older adults are simply the most sedentary segment of the population. The behavioural studies indicate that it is difficult to change two behaviours simultaneously. But it is easier to change one, especially the eating patterns and related behaviours. The activity related behaviour, on the other hand, may show inertia for change.

The ideology apart, health is the prime instrument that lets us enjoy life. The preservation of health is the best formula for longevity. A healthy food, adequate physical activity and wholesome lifestyle keep the daily attrition-related damage at minimum and retard ageing. An optimal healthcare adds further. An individual's life course may appear unpredictable, but it is not. The genetic and environmental factors, both being of equal importance, and behavioural patterns can successfully predict the life expectancy. The longer life is not separate from ageing slowly. They are mutually related.

The life is an eternal truth. We are because we live. We find people ageing; we ourselves age and grow older. The phenomenon of ageing is universal in the kingdom of living. With time, all living beings age. Yet, ageing is an enigma. We do not understand it. We do not exactly know, what makes us age and grow old, finally losing vitality of life? Living a healthy and long life is a common dream. All of us nourish the dream; all of us wish to realize it. But various disorders and infirmities annihilate the dream. Falling prey to them, we lose our health and fitness, and pass through an abridged life.

There have been immense developments in scientific research, including medical science. There has evolved a whole novel understanding of the biology of ageing. A vast body of knowledge can explain the changes that take place with ageing at molecular and cellular level. At the same time, the progress in healthcare and technology makes it possible to slow ageing. The science has progressed and there are futuristic visions of achieving significant longevity. There are possibilities of being able to reverse the ageing process. The eternal dream of immortality is on the verge of becoming a reality.

This book aims to provide answers to the questions related to ageing. It aims to explain ageing and charts out a program for slowing ageing. It also gives a peep into the futuristic visions of longevity and suggests scientific ways for a long life. Simultaneously, it is designed to educate you for fitness and to lead a healthy life. As you read through the book, you will find long-held views interspersed with shattering myths, and scientific facts intermingled with results from research and studies, which are still not out of the lab doors.

It may seem at times, but the book is not a fiction. Neither it is a concocted dream. The book is based on current state of scientific knowledge and gerontological research. I intend to share with you the current state of knowledge relating to ageing and gerontology. There are, to share with you, the facts and visions more eloquent than imaginations, and amazing thoughts amounting to the reality-pregnant-early-morning dreams.

You will notice few things as you read through the book. Using certain words has been avoided. You will only rarely find the words like aged, old, etc. The words like elderly have been used very sparingly. This has been done purposely and is well in line with the central thought of the book, which is to come out of our age-old prejudices against the old age.

So, I request you to read on. After all, theme of the book ageing slowly and living longer, as indicated by the title chosen, is of the prime concern to all of us. This book is a freshly edited and fully updated version of my book with the similar title first published in 2006, which was well appreciated by public as well as the scientific community world over.

August 15, 2020

Dr Vinod Nikhra M.D.

Contents

Contents

Contents

Contents

PART ONE

<u>LIVING AND AGEING</u>

CHAPTER ONE

THE ETERNAL DREAM:
Living a long life

FINITE LIFE, INFINITE DREAMS

Though not fixed, the lifespan of organisms, including human beings, is limited. As an organism, we go through the phases of birth, maturation, youth, ageing and death. We are born with unlimited potential. We grow to develop visions and dreams, which we look forward to realize. But meanwhile ageing slows us down. The ageing, which is universal in the kingdom of living. We find people ageing; we ourselves age and grow older. The ageing affects virtually all organs of the body and all parts of our social existence. As a social-being, we err many times; as a biological-being, we go on accumulating damage caused to body tissues due to disease processes and unhealthy lifestyles. In due course of time, the ageing takes its toll culminating as premature demise as the merciless death defaces the brief existence.

The socio-economic development and advances in healthcare have improved the life expectancy at birth and lifespan, in general. The vision of a lengthy-healthy life is alluring, but a possibility now, and holds promise to let enjoy the life at fullest. Here, in this beautiful world, the inanimate wonders compete with those animate to amaze us. The daily rising sun and cool moonlight never fail to excite us. The chirping of birds tickles our mind. The early morning breeze enlivens your heart; the falling night calms it. Listening to Louis Armstrong[1], you think '*What A Wonderful World* it is'. The life awakens so many dreams and giveth chance to fulfil. Living is such a joyful experience, and more so if life is not finite.

THE ESSENCE OF LIFE

People do similar things for different reasons. In the same way, each of us lives the life for different reasons. Some look forward to amassing wealth and fame. Some live for their loved ones. There can be a long list of such reasons. But in the essence, we live because the life gives us joy. Primarily, we are because we live. Living the life, gives a meaning to it. Life gone, there is no world for you.

Let us not dilute the issues. All things apart, living is itself the objective. This is well demonstrated by all powerful survival instinct percolating through the bio-spora. Meaning does not grant life, but life finds the meaning. In fact, life is never enough. The more you live, more you cherish. By living, you find your people and things. You make connections. You weave a world, a world of your creation, in which you want to live for forever. This is the prime thing, the eternal dream.

LONG LIFE AND AGEING

All of us want to lead a healthy and long life. But there are some requisites. A healthy body imparts the capability to lead an independent life and enjoy the living. Each of us has so many things to do. In fact, they emerge and enlarge as we live through the life. We do not plan to age; it just comes by to make us infirm. The long life and ageing are not contradictory. In fact, the ageing is just a temporal notion, which need not disable you. Here, thus, comes the concept of a healthy or successful ageing, which will make living significantly longer possible. We should plan for a healthy ageing.

THE ISSUES OF AGEING

There come certain kinds of issues, when we consider the phenomenon of ageing. The first concerns the ageing in terms of length of time. The second issue is that of functional problems afflicting the ageing individuals. The older adults may develop disability or incapacity for independent living. This occurs as the result of damage load due to pre-existing diseases or due to the ageing process itself, or both. The third kind of issue occurs at a more sublime level and involves behavioral attitudes and prejudices in the individuals themselves or prevalent in the society. A child, a youth or an older adult, all have equal right to live and look forward to a better living. There need not exist any prejudice against those older in age. The life force need not be diluted at any phase.

THE DREAM
COMING TRUE

In essence, ageing is a disorder of accumulated recurrent injury at molecular and cellular levels. The developmental factors leading to the damage load in early phases of life complicate the injury further[2]. These factors have a bearing on the residual functional capacity and cannot be taken as separate from the ageing process. The remedial measures, thus, need essentially cover the structural and functional loss due three types of damages: the developmental damage load, damaging effects of early life situations, and adverse effects of chronic disease processes.

The advanced research in gerontology holds promise. We can look forward to repairing the damages using gene technology, rejuvenative medication and futuristic nano-biotechnology. Mitigating the damaging effects of various factors, through a careful and healthy lifestyle and optimal healthcare, meanwhile, can help in slowing down the ageing process.

CHAPTER TWO

THE ETERNAL QUEST:
'Le Yayati Syndrome'

LOSS OF LIFE FORCE AND REMORSE

We live through the life along a line. From being born to infancy and childhood, the phases of adolescence and youth, the stages of adulthood and middle age, and the elder-hood and final phase of old age. Each stage leads to next one, often without a gross demarcation and before we can realize. The later ones often come to us as a shock.

One day we are pushed to the realization that we do not belong to the world of youth, when newer generation start distancing and knitting their flimsy world to increasingly exclude us. The process of losing relevance with the current world, thus, sets in. In time, with diminished life force, there occurs gradual loss of vigour. With losing something, which we once owned and took for granted, lets down the eternal truth of impermanence of life upon us.

'Le YAYATI SYNDROME'

The Yayati syndrome can be said to exist when there is a wish, amounting to a yearning, for youthfulness when one is on the verge of losing it or has already lost it.

The human lifespan may seem long when we compare it with that of other organisms. When we are child, we want to grow up as the adulthood seems a stage when one can make his or her own independent decisions. The various efforts, playing, learning and education, prepare you for the all-important adulthood. The adulthood comes with independence and power, independence about oneself and often with power on others. Then, everyone has a unique dream about his life carrying on a special notion about oneself.

There comes the nascent adulthood with all its joys, stresses and turmoil. The life goes with an accelerated pace. Years pass before one can count them. Enjoy the life we do, but the vagaries of life take their own toll on the phases of life. Soon passes the youthfulness, leaving its imprints on the human psyche. Realizing the gradual loss, there dawns an acute feeling of despair, there arise the yearnings to hold back the youthfulness and find the state of non-ageing.

THE STORY OF YAYATI

Let us recall the story from Indian mythology. Yayati, the ancient king, was cursed to become prematurely old. Yayati got the old age, which destroyed his handsomeness. He suffered with misery of sudden loss of youth, accentuated by pangs of recollection of his youthfulness. But he could exchange this for a young man's youth. He begged all his sons to exchange his old age for their youth. One son, Puru, agreed. When the delighted Yayati embraced Puru, the transfer was complete. Puru became a ripe old man in the prime of his youth while king Yayati regained his youth.

Yayati pursued pleasure and merriment with a renewed zest. The more he indulged, the thirstier he grew. In due course of time the truth dawned on him. In his words, told to Puru, 'Dear son, sensual desire is never quenched by indulgence any more than fire is by pouring oil on it. No object of desire, nothing can ever satisfy the desire of man. We can find peace only by a mental poise that goes beyond likes and dislikes.' With these words Yayati took back his old age. Puru, who regained his youth, was made king by Yayati, who retired to the forest to perform penance.

LESSONS FROM YAYATI

We should take down the Story of Yayati with the usual caution associated with mythological tales. The mythology thrives on dramatism and moral teachings. Never-the-less, few things stand out -

Firstly, it is in the human nature, perhaps a biological attribute, that the sensual things and worldly joys attract us all. Many times, they give us an apparent meaning to our life. Often, they are too powerful and drift us from moral code and socially acceptable behaviour. In the case of Yayati, taking the youth from his son, Puru, is example of this trait.

Secondly, as we mature, we grow over the joy of sensual indulgence, realizing the folly of it. In due course of time, we find alternatives that refurbish the meaning to life. With this intellectual growth, there grows our vision of life, now enclosing a larger world and its welfare in our purview.

And, thirdly, for the joy of indulgence we trade-off our social position and advantage, and lose on our health. The sex as an act and life course are interrelated. It is proved by scientific research that a relative celibacy may enhance longevity. We will learn more on this issue in later chapters.

IMPORTANCE
OF BEING YAYATI

There is a Yayati in all of us. In due course of time, seeing the loss of our youthfulness, the yearnings infect us too. Taking to Viagra is just an aspect of the Yayati syndrome. Being on brink of losing something we possessed earlier and enjoyed, and the recollection of those joyful moments, often decide our behavioural patterns.

The youthfulness, over-indulgence and dawn of wisdom, too, are the events along the lifeline. The concept of joy, changes all through our life. For a child a toy gives joy, for an adult it is something different. With maturity, we enjoy power, which now drives us. In due course of time, though, we grow to newer needs with advancing age.

SCIENTIFIC VISIONS IN THE STORY

The story of Yayati reads like a sci-fi. The dramatic effects, like, curses are usual in mythology. But, here – 'the transfer was complete. Puru became a ripe old man… while Yayati regained his youth' – and 'Yayati took back his old age. Puru, who regained his youth' – point to the fact that in those ancient days these things could have been possible. We are making amazing discoveries of modern times, but perhaps they existed but lost to us somehow.

Anyway, the story points us to the possibility of similar visions of healthy longevity and state of non-ageing in future. The gerontological and anti-ageing research is fast advancing. The dreams of today may become realm of tomorrow.

CHAPTER THREE

THE ETERNAL DILEMMA:
Finite and Ageing

THE PLASICITY OF LIFESPAN

An organism's lifespan is limited, so is of the human-being. Some may think that the brevity does give joy to life. But this, nihilism, seems improper. The life is a celebration. We do not celebrate brevity and demise. The joy comes not with quitting, but in enduring. At the biological level, the root factors, which evolve the protective mechanism called the survival instinct, endorse the fact that the evolution has prepared us for longevity, not the brevity.

To stay alive is our basic biological drive and attribute. It is a natural precondition for all other activities. Today, a period of about 30,000 days is the average human lifespan. For a centenarian, it is about 40,000 days. The things are better at present. Two centuries back, as per the data, the life expectancy in 1796, was around 10,000 days, but doubled a century later. A little while ago, the average life expectancy was less than 20 years or about 7,000 days[3]. Thus, the human lifespan though finite, is not fixed. It can be moulded gradually into a more favourable one.

THE BIOLOGY OF DECAY AND REPAIR

Whereas ageing may mean decaying, as the repairing process falters, the living means restoring and rejuvenating the body tissues and organs. But at some phase in life, living becomes ageing. According to the Reliability theory, widely applied in engineering and now being applied to explain ageing, with time the ageing system falters, leading to the failure unless the cause is corrected or the faltering parts are renewed and replaced.

The ageing process, thus, contributes to the age-related gradual decline in functional threshold, performance, productivity and health (Fig 2).

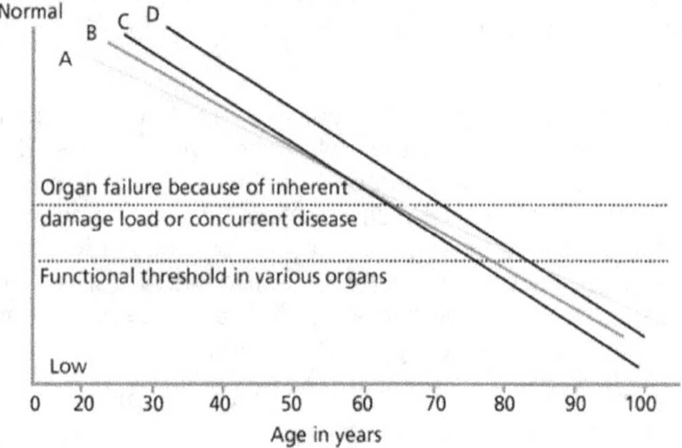

Figure 2: Age-related decline in functional threshold, performance and productivity.

There are three main causes of decay: disease, trauma and ageing. Looking at the brighter side, a number of advances in healthcare seem to have gradually nullified the deterioration due to most of the diseases, infectious as well as non-infectious. The ageing, representing a collection of cumulative changes at the molecular and cellular level, is not an event. Thus, we do not age all of a sudden, rather it comes gradually. Hence, the ageing can be regarded as a process made of various components. As we, go on understanding the components of ageing and developing the means to correct them, we win over the biological decay in steps.

THE ILL-FOUNDED QUALMS AND FEARS

All of us, an optimist or a pessimist, fear ageing. An optimist lives through the life with hope of finding a way that will cure or at least to delay the ageing. Whereas the pessimist has lost all the hopes and seems to be suffering with a kind of chronic disorder of melancholy or hopelessness.

No wonder, a ray of hope or even a reminiscence of lost times when longevity was possible excites us. 'Lost Horizon', a novel by James Hilton, published in 1933, was a huge success. In it, the hero finds inner peace, love, and a sense of purpose in fictional town, Shangri-La, whose inhabitants also enjoy longevity. The book has inspired countless travels to discover Shangri-La, two films and names of places around the world.

The ageing issues concern the ageing in terms of length of time as well as relate to the functional aspect with the older adults developing disability or incapacity for independent living as the result of damage load due to pre-existing diseases or due to the ageing process itself. Rationalizing, it may be apparent that the fears about old age and reaction to those fears are ill-founded. Many scientists and researchers now believe that, for the first time in human history, we have come close to understanding the basic characteristics of human ageing and possible ways to defeat it. It appears that the ageing represents a failure-prone mechanism, which can be improved, corrected, and better maintained through scientific interventions.

THE CONFUSION AND CONTRADICTIONS

We live and age in a time full of paradox. On one hand, people consider the ageing process as something inevitable and invincible often doubting the promising findings of anti-ageing research. On the other hand, we witness them practicing various anti-ageing measures themselves, from following healthy lifestyles to preserve the body to applying anti-wrinkle cream and lotion.

But the dilemma is not a simple confusion but a contradiction of notions. It represents the crisis of long-held views, as the novel research challenges the old stereotypes. It also indicates that the notions of possibility of winning over the ageing are making inroads into our life. Hence, it is a welcome event.

Understanding biological basis of the ageing process has led to insights that are able to potentially identify measures to slow down the aging process. The ageing, thus, becomes a modifiable risk factor and there are expectant possibilities to extend the lifespan and improve health-span.

Through targeted lifestyle changes and potentially effective interventions through nutraceuticals and pharmaceuticals, and stem cell therapy, it may be possible to reduce the age-related chronic and debilitating morbidities and improve the health-span.

FROM AGEING SLOWLY TO EXPONENTIAL LIFE EXTENSION AND IMMORTALITY

CLARKE'S THIRD LAW

With advances in gerontology, there has evolved a whole novel understanding of the biology of ageing. The ageing is a complex process and affects virtually all organs of the body. A vast body of knowledge can now explain the changes that take place with ageing at molecular and cellular level. But irrational hopes from technology move us away from terra-ferma and are detrimental to rational scientific behaviour. Thinking rationally, it is unlikely that something like a pill or potion, can reverse the changes and dysfunction associated with ageing. At the same time, the progress in healthcare and technology has made possible to slow ageing. Further, there are possibilities of being able to reverse the ageing process.

As the life expectancy at birth rises and there is taking place an improvement in average and maximum lifespan, the possibility of living life more than never before seems logical. The science gives visions; the technology makes the visions possible. The future technology appears to offer us visions that rival the dreams of myth and legend. As per the Arthur C. Clarke's Third Law[4], 'any sufficiently advanced technology is indistinguishable from magic'. One of these magical dreams is that of exponential life extension.

REGENERATIVE MEDICINE AND QUEST FOR IMMORTALITY

Apart from caloric restriction (CR), the regenerative medicine is the next concrete step for achieving longevity. The most promising in regenerative medicine is the therapeutic cloning. A new organ can be grown for transplantation using one's own cells. The process would involve transferring the nucleus from a cell to an enucleated human egg, which would then grow to the blastocyst stage. Stem cells would be harvested from the blastocyst and transformed into the desired tissues for transplant. The regenerative medicine aims higher, it does not retard or slow ageing but corrects the organ failure and diseases that accompany ageing. It is an advanced form of future science.

Finally, the life is not a myth but an eternal truth. We are because we live. Living a healthy and long life is a common dream. All of us nourish the dream; all of us wish to realize it. Various diseases and infirmity annihilate the dream. Falling prey to ageing we lose our health and fitness and pass through an abridged life. Scientifically speaking, the longer life is not separate from ageing slowly, rather they are mutually related. With the scientific progress the futuristic visions of achieving significant longevity, if not immortality, seem quite possible. Of course, the likelihood of the impact of exponential survival cannot be foreseen in totality. The eternal dream of exponential healthy life extension is on the verge of becoming a reality[5].

PART TWO

<u>BIOLOGY OF AGEING</u>

CHAPTER FOUR

LIFESPAN AND EVOLUTION:
Determinants of Ageing

THE LIFE-FORMS AND LIFESPAN

Under the socio-cultural layers, we human beings are biological organisms and share the same fate like other members of the bio-spora. The lifespan of organisms is limited, though not fixed. An organism goes through the phases of life, birth, maturity, ageing and death. The reproduction, whether sexual or asexual, allows new organisms to replace the old ones. Thus, continues the uninterrupted cycle of life.

Further, as the new organisms replace in time the older-ones, and adapt to the changes in echo-sphere, the process allows evolution to take place. The phenomenon is going on through the Millennia. The advantageous changes are passed on to the next generation, the deleterious ones are eliminated along with the organism in due course of time. And, thus, goes on the incessant evolution.

Is it through the evolution process, that the Mother Nature limits life span of an organism? Different organisms have different life spans. The microscopic roundworm, Caenorhabditis elegans, has a lifespan of about 3 weeks, a mouse of about 3 years, bats of about 20 years, and humans can live for about 100 years. The plants live longer, many surviving to hundreds of years, still not showing changes related to ageing. But, some simple organisms, such as amoeba and hydra, have an indefinite life span, apparently free of an intrinsic senescence.

THE BIOLOGICAL AGEING CLOCK

Is there something inherent in the anatomy or physiology of lifeforms that limits the lifespan? Does there exist a biological ageing clock? Perhaps, not. The Mother Nature is not our enemy. It is not against longevity. Rather it tries to promote a long life. The organisms are not programmed to die, but to survive the adversities that they may encounter. Even the programmed cell death, an intrinsic phenomenon occurring at cellular level called apoptosis, is a mechanism that is meant to favour survival of the whole organism.

Thus, there does not exist a biological ageing clock limiting survival. But things do happen randomly, like accidents, diseases, and environmental adversities, which affect to deteriorate health or set in the damage at tissue, organ, or systemic level, and may accentuate the ageing.

GENETIC INFLUENCE ON LIFESPAN

Whether the genes have a bearing on the life span? The answer seems, yes. The studies among twins indicate that monozygotic twins have a more similar life span than heterozygotic twins, leading to the assumption that there is some inheritability of chances of longevity from parents to children. Experimentally also, it has been shown that genetic mutations influence the life span of organisms.

The genes are, thus, important. They decide the body appearance, structure and functioning of inner organs, metabolism, oxidative stress, immunity and even working of psyche including the intelligence quotient. They have impact on ageing process and predispose to various diseases, as well. In simple organisms like C. elegans, a nematode, the genes through DAF-2 and DAF-16 transcription factors and signaling pathways, have been shown to influence ageing (Fig 3).

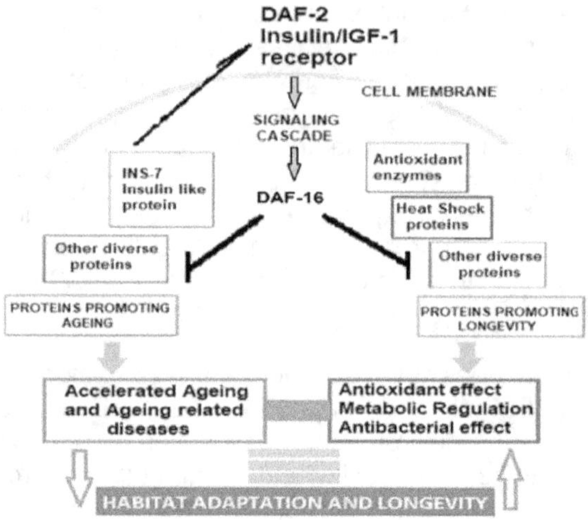

Figure 3: IGF and insulin signalling pathway and DAF-2 and DAF-16 transcription factors in C. elegans influencing ageing.

But whether do they solely control ageing? Probably not, otherwise, there would have been no great variation in the lifespan among individuals of the same species. The studies also show that the genes account only for about one-fourth of what determines the life span and other factors including environmental and certain random events have a bearing on three-fourths of the lifespan[6].

REPRODUCTIVE ISSUES: SEX AND CELIBACY

The life is birth, growth, reproduction, ageing, death, and evolution through generations. The reproduction is what through which the Mother Nature replaces the new for the old. Thinking other way round, whether the factors like sex and reproduction have a bearing on the ageing process and life span?

The studies show that unmated fruit flies live longer than those, which mate. In females, perhaps, the egg laying process imposes a survival cost. Also, species with smaller litter sizes as compared to their own body size tend to survive longer. Further, in a particular species, the body size may influence the ageing and survival. The much-debated human study – the aristocrat study – which compared the number of children and the age at which the mothers had their first child, and related these values with the age at death, is important in this context. The study inferred those women who reached an older age and a higher life span, delivered less children and at a later age[7].

But what is the relevant issue true about the males? Does celibacy improve the chances of survival, or the virility affects it adversely? Whether a low-profile sex life is associated with longevity? The folklores link celibacy, absolute or relative, with a reduced incidence of infirmity associated with ageing and a longer life. Whether the layman-belief about seminal conservation has some scientific basis or just a modified version of leading a balanced life? These are certain issues, not studied in detail so far and hence, presently, the science fails to provide a definite answer.

STRESS OF LIVING AND BIOLOGICAL ATTRITION

As we live through our life, we are exposed to oxidative and other stresses, leading to attrition and biological damage at tissue levels. We accumulate wastes and toxins, which our bodies are unable to get rid of. There occur some changes in our genome due to inner causes like mitochondrial generation of free radicals and external factors like cosmic radiations. Every time a cell divides, there is the potential for error. Oxidative stress is also a potential source of damage at molecular level. Free radicals are generated within mitochondria and have potential to alter the cellular material and internal structures. Through p53, the guardian of genome and another protein p21, these factors have been linked with senescence and living span at the cellular level, and the organ reserve and redundancy affecting ageing and its fallouts.

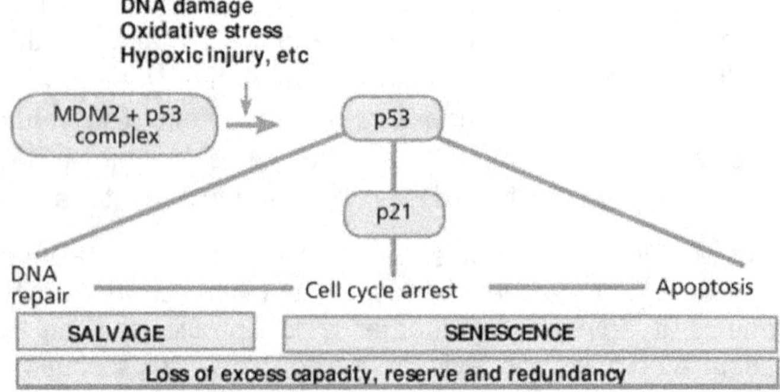

Figure 4. Oxidative stress, DNA damage and ageing link

The damage at molecular and cellular levels, and the process of faltered repair, thus, influence the ageing process (Fig 4). The cells possess a number of systems for functional and structural maintenance and repair. In fact, the DNA-repair capability correlates well with the lifespan of a species. Also, there is a correlation between the ability to respond to stress and the life span. An increased stress resistance has been noted in long-lived genetic strains. The much talked about cells of today, the stem cells have a higher resilience than the well-differentiated cells.

THE FOOD, AGEING AND LIFESPAN

The food and dietary patterns have a bearing on ageing and the life span. By and large, the diet influences the life expectancy. The studies show that in the nematode, C. elegans, a mutation of the genes involved in the insulin-signaling pathway, namely daf2 and daf16 genes can induce an up to 2-fold increase in life span. The caloric restriction also influences the life expectancy and ageing.

Thus, several external, behavioral, and internal factors influence ageing, life span, and quality of life during lifespan. These include the environment, genetic inheritance, sex and reproduction, food and dietary style, the accumulation of cellular attrition and damage, and the inherent ability to repair. No doubt, the process of ageing begins much earlier than usually thought.

CHAPTER FIVE

THE OVERVIEW OF AGEING:
Changes Associated with Ageing

THE WEAR AND TEAR CHANGES

There occur anatomical and physiological alterations in human body with the age. The time takes a toll on the organs and systems in the body. It is like a wear and tear process and how and when this occurs is unique to an individual. As such, the ageing can be called an inter-play of genome and the environment. There occur typical natural changes with the age involving heart and blood vessels, skin and muscles, teeth, bones and joints, digestive organs and kidneys, nerves, sensory organs and brain, and ovaries and uterus in women and testes and prostate in men. Essentially all body organs and systems are involved in ageing process to a significant or lesser extent.

The main reason we are concerned about ageing is because it is related to health deterioration and increased morbidity. The health deterioration takes place in some earlier whereas in comes later in others. The same is true for life span; some live longer whereas others do not. Thus, the clinical medicine and bio-gerontology are interrelated.

THE EXTERNAL CHANGES

The wrinkles and gray hair are obvious changes we notice with one growing older. These are the external changes. These are the signs by which we can guess somebody's age. But the age and extent of the external changes differs from person to person. Thus, some appear to look to age early, whereas others stay looking youthful. The wrinkles and grey hair may come early or may appear late.

• Skin, nails, and hair

With age, the skin becomes thin, less elastic and more fragile. It bruises more easily. Decreased production of natural oils makes the skin drier and more wrinkled. Age spots and skin tags occur.

The nails grow at a slow pace. The hair becomes thin and gray. An older adult perspires less. The ageing changes in skin depend on many factors including the exposure to sun, smoking, etc.

• Teeth

Broadly speaking, the teeth and gums respond to age depending on how well they have been cared over the years. With advancing age, mouth feels drier, gums recede, teeth darken and become more brittle. With less saliva to wash away bacteria the teeth and gums become vulnerable to decay and infection. Dry mouth also makes speaking slow, swallowing difficult and tasting poor.

• Weight and Height

With age, the metabolism generally slows down, meaning that the body now burns fewer calories. Calories that were once used to meet daily energy needs instead are stored as fat. The overall level of activity may decrease, resulting in unwanted weight gain. There occurs some decrease in the height because of decreased muscular tone and osteoporotic bone changes

THE INTERNAL CHANGES

But what is exactly going on inside the body with age, is much more Important. As we age, the time takes its toll on the organs and systems in our body. The internal changes, in a way, may be, considered as a wear and tear injury. But the rate at which this occurs is unique to a person. The ageing changes in the organs include:

• Heart and blood vessels

With ageing the heart muscle becomes a less efficient pump. Hardened fatty deposits (atherosclerosis) narrow the arterial lumens. The natural loss of elasticity, in combination with atherosclerosis, makes arteries stiffer and less elastic, increasing the work load on the heart. The changes affect the heart functioning and blood supply, and can cause high blood pressure and enlargement of heart, and lead to heart failure in due course of time.

With age, there is decrease in pacemaker cells resulting in a slowing of heart rate but the blood pumping function is maintained by increasing the volume of the blood pumped out. In addition, there is decreased responsiveness to adrenergic receptor stimulation, a decreased reactivity to baroreceptors and chemoreceptors and an increase in circulating adrenaline like hormones. The ageing changes in heart and vasculature, being important issue, are described in a latter chapter.

• Bones, muscles, and joints
The bones reach their maximum mass between ages 25 and 35. Later, with age, they shrink in size and density. The gradual loss of density weakens the bones and makes them susceptible to fracture. Muscles, tendons and joints, also, lose strength and flexibility with age.

• Digestive system
The swallowing of food becomes cumbersome and the propulsion of the digested food through the intestines slows down with age. The amount of surface area within intestines diminishes. Also, the flow of secretions from stomach, liver, pancreas, and small intestine decrease. But these changes generally do not disrupt digestive processes. The constipation is often the first noticeable digestive symptom with ageing.

• Kidneys and urogenital system

With age, the kidneys become less efficient in filtering the waste. Certain chronic diseases like diabetes and high blood pressure, damage kidneys further. About 30 percent of older adults suffer with loss of bladder control, called urinary incontinence. The pelvic muscles become weaker with ageing, reducing bladder support. Incontinence can also be caused by obesity, frequent constipation, and chronic cough.

Women are more likely to suffer from urinary incontinence than men. The post-menopausal women may experience stress incontinence as the muscles around the opening of the bladder, the sphincter muscles, reduce in volume and lose strength with declining gonadal hormones. In older men, incontinence may be caused by an enlarged prostate, which can block the urethra. This causes difficulty in emptying bladder and small amounts of urine may leak out.

• Brain and nervous system

Loss of brain cells or neurons is a natural part of the ageing process. Starting at around age 30, the human brain begins to lose neurones at rate of roughly five to ten percent per decade. This loss of brain tissue affects various functions, including memory, understanding, and decision-making. However, the loss neurons in the brain or outside is attended by increase in number of connections between the remaining neurons increases, to compensate for the loss and ageing neurons to maintain brain function. The reflexes tend to become slower and there may develop in-coordination.

The memory becomes less efficient in older adults, who may lose the ability to bank new memories. Some older people may manifest lack attention span to log new information into their memory, when the brain's attention center in the prefrontal cortex is primarily involved. Those having a significant memory problem may be suffering from Mild Cognitive Impairment (MCI) - a condition causing them to forget the details of conversations and upcoming appointments, but still allows them to function independently, drive, manage their money, etc. But those with MCI are at risk for developing Alzheimer's disease. The ageing changes in brain and nerves, being important issue, are described in a latter chapter.

• Sensory organs

With age, there is less tear formation. The retinas thin and lenses gradually turn yellow and become less clear. In focusing on near objects becomes difficult. Later, the irises stiffen, making the pupils less responsive. This makes difficult to adapt to different levels of light. Cataracts, glaucoma and macular degeneration are the common problems associated with ageing

Hearing loss is a common condition affecting older adults. One in three persons older than 60 and half of all those older than 85 have significant hearing loss. In addition, the walls of auditory canals thin, and eardrums thicken. There may be difficulty in hearing high frequency sounds. To follow a conversation in a crowded room may be difficult.

CHAPTER SIX

PSYCHOSOCIAL HEALTH:
Spirituality, Intimacy and Sex

SPIRITUAL HEALTH:
POSITIVITY AND TRANQUILITY

We can never escape from the stress of daily living. The stress is a reality of life, more so because the world is becoming more and more complex. In simple words, the stress is something you perceive, strain is the harm it does to your body and psyche. We cannot simply turn back to the olden times. But we can positively manage stress and allay the harmful strain.

We can solve the complexity of life by creating an island of simplicity. This will entail creation of a tranquil life in the midst of the complex world. Certain simple acts like attending a place of worship or owning a pet have been linked to a longer life. Simultaneously, following a healthy and balanced lifestyle will help in keeping the stress at minimum.

One of the common observations is that those who live long are optimistic. They may differ in body type and habitat, but they have been mostly healthy during their life. This may be dependent on a balanced hormonal state of well-being. The brain, too, masters the vital functions through hormones and neural networks. The ageing may be controlled by a gamut of programs in our brains. In worms, the life span is favourably regulated by a hibernation cycle. In humans, sleep is the closest thing to hibernation.

THE NEED OF INTIMATE
RELATIONSHIP

With age, sexual needs, patterns and performance may change. The older adults are active and continue to do many of the things they enjoyed during their younger years. This includes enjoying sex and intimate relationships. In fact, the studies show that most individuals still have sexual fantasies and desires well into their 60s and 70s, if not later. A healthy sexual relationship is a part of good physical health.

The need for intimate relationship does not dilute with age. The need for affection, emotional closeness and intimate love persists in the later years. But, ageing as such, definitely affects the sexuality. As the body ages, there occur certain changes affecting the sexual relationships and ability to perform and maintain intimacy with the partner. There also takes place a psychological re-makeup.

PHYSIOLOGICAL CHANGES AFFECTING INTIMACY

The hormone, testosterone, regulates the sex drive in both, men and women. Most of the ageing men and women produce enough testosterone to maintain their interest in sex. But there take place certain changes with the age, affecting aspects of sexual life.

• Women: With menopause and reduced estrogen levels, there is a reduced lubrication and loss of inherent elasticity of female organ. These two changes may make the sex less comfortable or even painful during the later years.

• Men: With age, a man may take longer to achieve an erection. The latter may be less firm and may not last as long. Ageing also increases the time interval between possible erections.

ERECTILE DYSFUNCTION IN MAN

The prevalence and severity of erectile dysfunction (ED) increase with advancing age. According to Massachusetts Male Ageing Study the proportion of subjects with severe ED increased from 5 percent at the age of 40 years to 15 percent at the age of 70 years[8].

There are multiple factors contributing to age-related ED:

• The relational factors are important in older adults. The loss of interest in the partner or decrease in partner's sexual interest can be related to reduced sexual activity at all ages. The embarrassment about the sexual needs as an older adult can also affect the ability to perform. Appearance of wrinkles and gray hair may lead to a poor body image, affecting the emotional ability to connect. A poor body image can reduce the sex drive. The stress can lead to performance anxiety and can trigger impotence in men.

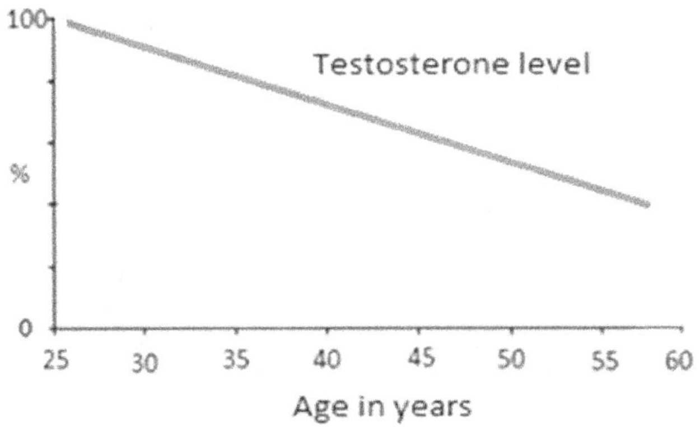

Figure 5: Ageing and testosterone level in men

• The age-related changes in endocrine function can cause ED in older adults (Fig 5). Testosterone levels decline with age, though there is no definite correlation between testosterone level and the severity of ED. Some older adult males reporting hypoactive sexual desire may have significantly lower testosterone levels.

• Chronic diseases like, coronary heart disease, high blood pressure, peripheral vascular disease and metabolic diseases, like diabetes can cause a significant sexual dysfunction. Certain degenerative neurological disease such Parkinson's and Alzheimer's disease can lead to ED.

• The association of depression and ED is controversial. There appears to be a link between depression and ED. The prevalence of depressive disorders increases progressively with age until the age of about 60 years, then it remains stable in the following 15-20 years, and increasing again only later.

• Some medications can contribute to ED. The drugs such as antidepressants and antipsychotic; anti-hypertensive, those used for coronary heart disease and prokinetic drugs have been associated with ED. The age-dependent increase in the use of these medications may play an important role. ED can be associated with prostate surgery.

MEASURES FOR SEXUAL HEALTH IN OLDER ADULTS

Many older adults find that their sex life deteriorate as they age. The embarrassment in discussing sexual problems is common. But conversations with the doctor will help in understanding the changes.

Improving sex life may require certain changes in the outlook and technique:

• Expanding the definition of sex: The sexual life encompasses something sublime than the intercourse. With the age, other options may be more comfortable and more fulfilling.

- Communicating with the partner: Discussing about the changes one is going through and one's changing needs and likes also helps.

- Changing the routine: Some simple tips can help in improving the sex life during later years. Changing the time of day, a longer foreplay and a new sexual position may help.

- Managing one's expectations: Do not expect to have lots of sex as an older adult. One can express intimacy with the partner in other ways, as well.

- Taking care and keeping fit: A healthy diet and a regular exercise keep the body fit. Excess alcohol should be avoided.

SEX NEEDS OF SINGLE OLDER ADULTS

The older adults, who are single, also need an intimate relationship and look forward to it. It is never too late to start a new relationship. Meeting new people and going to new places will help. Meeting a new person may lead to friendship and intimate relationship in due course of time.

PART THREE

<u>UNDERSTANDING AGEING</u>

CHAPTER SEVEN

AGEING AND DISEASE:
Accompaniments of Ageing

The ageing and disease process complicate each other. With ageing the residual power of tissues and organ declines. Simultaneously, there is a decline in activities associated with daily living. These two factors modify the manifestations of various diseases. The underlying diseases and disorders, when present, may accelerate ageing process and the complications due to ageing worsen the clinical course of illness.

THE AGEING OF SKIN

The skin ages as we grow older. Lax and wrinkled skin is synonymous with the old age. The effort at ageing slowly, thus, means a quest for youthful skin also. But the ageing changes in skin can also be viewed as a protective phenomenon, whereby the tissue loses its maximal functionality and reserve capacity but also protects itself against potential mutations that may result in cancer.

One of the DNA changes that are part of the ageing response is progressive telomere shortening as cells continue to divide. Finally, the telomeres are lost and the cell that cannot divide any further enters in senescence phase. Exposure of skin to ultraviolet rays may accelerate the shortening of telomeres, pushing cells into senescence. The melanin in skin serves as a shield protecting DNA. Thymidine dimers are produced when light damages DNA. In most instances, these are repaired by enzymes in the nucleus. However, cumulative and repetitive sun exposure may result in multiple sites of dimer formation, exceeding the ability of nuclear enzymes to repair the dimers. The UV-mediated effects on skin then become obvious.

Molecular Basis of Skin Ageing

Alterations in the composition of collagen in the dermis may play a role in wrinkling of aged skin. Light may be functioning as an inducer of certain enzymes, such as collagenase, which may result in damage to collagen molecules.

The UV exposure triggers activator proteins, which in turn increase expression of collagenase and decrease expression of procollagen. The reduction of procollagen may result in reduced amounts of healthy collagen in the dermis. This leads to 'micro-scars.' which may not be visible initially. Beyond a certain level of cumulative UV light-induced damage, the result of photo-ageing manifests as wrinkles.

Dealing with Skin Ageing

Retinoids help to restore procollagen in human skin by preventing increased collagenase expression. Skin from younger patients seems to have a collagen content equivalent to that of skin from older patients treated with topical retinoids.

The subcutaneous structures including fat, muscles, and dermis play an important role in giving the skin a younger look. This can be brought about by a process called subcutaneous tissue augmentation. The filing agents (for example, hyaluronic acid) are used for tissue augmentation.

Botulinum toxin is a useful adjunct in treatment of patients with moderate-to-severe ageing skin. The depressors can be treated by botulinum toxin. For horizontal forehead lines, a few injections followed by massage to the site can result in sufficient toxin spread. The orbicularis oculi muscle can be injected around the eye to make the eye appear bigger.

ANAEMIA AND AGEING

Identifying Anaemia

Diagnosing anemia is important because -

- Anemia may be the first sign of a serious underlying disease, such as cancer of the digestive system or vitamin B12 deficiency, that may be lethal if left undiagnosed, and
- Anemia is associated with and may partly be the cause of a number of morbid conditions, including functional dependence, dementia, renal failure, cardiac failure, etc.

According to the World Health Organization, anaemia is defined as a hemoglobin level of less than 13 g/dl in men and less than 12 g/dl in women. A number of physiologic findings support this definition. The secretion of erythropoietin is increased when hemoglobin levels fall below 12 g/dl, indicating that these levels of hemoglobin are necessary for optimal tissue oxygenation.

The prevalence of anaemia increases with age in older adults. Women are more susceptible to anemia at a younger age due to menstrual blood loss and childbearing iron loss, while men have a higher prevalence of anaemia-related morbidity at an older age.

The association of anaemia with age is of particular concern. Of special interest are the effects of anemia on survival, function and quality of life. It is important to find the cause of anemia in older individuals to establish the reversibility of this condition. There is possibility that correction of anemia might delay or reverse to some extent ageing itself.

Anaemia in Older Adults

The ageing by itself does not lead to anaemia. In older adults it is often due to increased prevalence of various diseases. As such, older adults become more vulnerable to anaemia when faced by hemopoietic stress. Ageing is associated with a progressive reduction in the functional reserve of various body organs.

The hemopoiesis, i.e. blood production, may become compromised by a number of factors including reduced number of hemopoietic stem cells with age, reduced sensitivity of stem cells, reduction of growth factors, and increased circulation of substances, like cytokines, that inhibit hemopoiesis. The qualitative changes in hemopoiesis may also occur with age and compromise the hemopoietic reserve.

A relative deficiency of erythropoietin may occur with age. Iron deficiency due to chronic blood loss from ulcers, piles, etc. may occur. Anemia of chronic disease, including chronic kidney disease, is probably the most common form of anemia in the elderly. A deficiency in vitamin B12 may occur in all elderly. In many cases, the cause of anemia may not be found. Here, the inadequate production of erythropoietin may be the cause.

**Clinical Implications
of Anaemia**

An appealing concept is the possibility that correction of anaemia may stop or slow down the ageing process and prevent ageing-related functional decline.

Survival: A number of studies have shown that anaemia is associated with a decreased survival rate in older adults. The risk of dying increases with the degree of anaemia. Alternatively, the risk of dying decreases when anaemia is corrected.

Fatigue and General Weakness: Fatigue is the most common symptom of anaemia. The causes of fatigue include energy imbalance and emotional distress. Anaemia is the most common cause of energy imbalance. Its correction results in improved energy levels. The prevention of fatigue reduces the functional dependence.

<u>Complications relating to heart and vessels</u>: Chronic anaemia may lead to enlargement of heart. In fact, every 1 gm/dl decrease in hemoglobin is associated with an increased incidence of heart enlargement by 6 percent. An enlarged heart is more likely to fail and associated with coronary heart disease.

<u>Anaemia and Cognition</u>: There is a correlation between anaemia and risk of MCI and Alzheimer disease. In fact, a number of cognitive and emotional complications, including headache, loss of concentration, and depression can occur.

<u>Risk of drug intolerance</u>: Anaemia increases the risk of adverse drug reactions by reducing the amount of drug that can be bound in blood. This, in turn, increases the concentration of free drug in circulation and also, by causing decreased oxygen in tissues, increases susceptibility.

AGEING, IMMUNITY AND CANCER

The primary function of immune system is to protect the organism from a variety of invasions and illnesses, including the development of cancer. But, various aspects of immunity change with advancing age. A major function of the immune system is to provide surveillance against the errant cells. There occurs an age-related decline in both the cellular and humoral components of the immune system. This decline leads to the accumulation of cellular and DNA mutations contributing to an increased incidence of cancers or malignancies.

Immunity at Cellular Level

T Lymphocytes

In ageing humans, there occurs involution of the thymus with ensuing loss of thymic hormones. Subsequently, changes in T lymphocytes are seen. The reactive T cells decline in number and the memory T cells increase. With advancing age, there is a loss of stem cell potential to generate T cells. The T-helper cells become less capable of generating cytotoxic effector cells to participate in delayed hypersensitivity reactions. As shown by *in vitro* studies, the suppressor cells from aged animals have handicap in recognizing and exerting suppressive effects against specific antigens from self and other agents.

B Lymphocytes

With increasing age, there is no change in the number of circulating B cells, but there take place structural changes in B-cell membranes and a decrease in numbers of bone marrow B-cell precursors. Simultaneously, the B cells ability to generate antibody response declines. The ability to respond to a new or previously encountered antigen challenge with specific antibody production is decreased with ageing.

Macrophages

One of the key constituents of the innate immune system are monocytes. There occur changes in the expression of functionally important cellular receptors on monocyte surface with ageing. This results in depressed chemotaxis and phagocytosis, as well as antigen processing and presentation, whereas cell activation and the secretion of inflammatory cytokines, such as IL-1, IL-6, TNF, are markedly increased.

Natural Killer Cells

Natural killer (NK) cells are cytotoxic cells that can act to destroy the targets without the need for antigen sensitization. Paradoxically, the number of NK cells increases with ageing, but NK activity decreases. Lymphokine-activated killer (LAK) cells, highly activated NK cells, are able to lyse certain cell lines that are resistant to NK cells. The activity of LAK cells also reduces with ageing.

Lymphocyte DNA

There is a high intra-individual variability between the levels of DNA damage in peripheral blood leucocytes. The significant factors that influence the DNA damage in leucocytes are age, sex and smoking habit[9]. There is an increased fragility of lymphocyte DNA with age, which predisposes to immuno-senescence.

Interleukins (ILs)

The activated T cells produce a variety of cell growth and differentiation factors. There is an age-related decline in lymphocyte production and response to other cytokines, such as IL-1, IL-2, etc. and tumor necrosis factor. The interleukins, IL-1 and IL-2, play a primary role in activation, recruitment, and proliferation of T lymphocytes. The studies indicate that older adults displaying a decline in absolute lymphocyte counts have higher mortality rates.

<u>Immune Control of Cancer</u>

The immune system protects the organism against the development of cancer by immune surveillance. It is constantly surveying for and eliminating a cancer as it arises at cellular level. Thus, the clinical cancer represents a failure of this system. The older adults with depressed immune function have a higher incidence rate and, indeed, the advanced age is the greatest risk factor for the development of cancer.

The incidence of cancers rises with age because those who live longer accumulate sequence of mutations, which ultimately result in development of a cancer. Normal age-related changes in susceptible tissues may lead to development of certain tumours such as the hormone-dependent cancers of breast, ovary, and endometrium, and that of prostate. However, though cancer incidence increases with age, the ageing changes in the biological systems may cause death much earlier before development of the malignancy.

PHYSIOLOGICAL AGEING AT CELLULAR LEVEL

• **Apoptosis:** The ageing process occurs at molecular and cellular level. It can be viewed as a process resulting from increased disorderliness of intra- and intercellular regulatory mechanisms. This disorderliness is also evident in the erosion of the orderly neuroendocrine feedback regulation of the secretion of growth hormone, luteinizing hormone, follicle-stimulating hormone, and adreno-corticotropin hormone.

At the cellular level, several processes are involved in the physiology of ageing and the development of ageing-related diseases. Apoptosis signifies the process of non-traumatic and non-inflammatory cell death that balances cell proliferation and thus maintains homeostasis. The specific gene products control, promoting and opposing, regulated cell death via mitochondrial effects. The deregulation of apoptosis has been implicated in the development of diseases that are more prevalent in older individuals, such as cancer and the neuro-degenerative disorders like Alzheimer's and Parkinson's diseases.

• **Telomere Shortening:** The short nucleotide sequences located on the ends of chromosomes also regulate the cellular senescence. Their length limits the number of possible cell divisions. The limited proliferative potential of cells is the result of the telomere shortening that occurs during DNA synthesis at each cell division. The extension of telomeres by the enzyme telomerase occurs in germ cells and cancerous cells and compensates for the loss of a few nucleotides of telomeric DNA during each cell cycle, essentially protecting and ensuring that the entire linear chromosome is completely replicated.

• **Oxidative Stress:** The reactive oxygen species (ROS) are produced as by-products of aerobic cellular metabolism and include free radicals such as superoxide anion ($O_2{\cdot}-$), hydroxyl radical ($\cdot OH$), as well as nonradical molecules like hydrogen peroxide (H_2O_2), singlet oxygen ($^1O_2$), and so forth. The ROS lead to recurrent and progressive oxidative injury in the ageing cells.

• **Other Factors:** The ageing-associated changes also occur between and among cells via alterations in the intercellular matrix, the intercellular exchange of trophic factors, the release of inflammatory cytokine mediators, and inflammatory or non-inflammatory infiltration by other cells.

THE AGE-RELATED HORMONAL CHANGES

The hormones are the chemical regulators for body composition - fat deposition, skeletal mass, muscle strength, metabolism and body weight, and physical well-being. Various alterations in general physique and physiology evolve with ageing and a number of these manifestations are related to the effects of declining hormone levels.

Ageing can be viewed as a variable process resulting from a disorderliness of regulatory mechanisms. It results in reduced robustness of the organism to concurrent stress and disease. There is the erosion of orderly neuroendocrine feedback regulation of the secretion of LH, FSH, ACTH, and GH. These physiological changes are manifested as menopause, andropause, adrenopause, and somatopause. This is attended by disruption of metabolic processes is associated with a higher prevalence of diseases such as type 2 diabetes and cancer in older individuals.

Further, in general, there is a remarkable variability in the physical status of ageing population. The ageing-related disorders like sarcopenia, osteopenia, and cognitive disorders, may reflect, in part, the natural polymorphisms of key gene products.

In humans, ageing is associated with a decrease in the production of estrogen in women, leading to menopause, and testosterone leading to andropause in men, dehydroepi-androsterone (DHEA) and DHEA sulphate in males leading to adrenopause; and a decrease in the activity of growth hormone (GH) and insulin-like growth factor (IGF) axis leading to somatopause.

The Ageing and Neuro-Endocrine Axis

The central nervous system regulates the pituitary gland, which in turn secretes hormones to act on target tissues. These hormones have a feedback mechanism through hypothalamus and pituitary. The gender markedly influences growth hormone (GH) secretion. The premenopausal women exhibit a 2-fold less rapid decline than men in daily GH production with increasing age. Withdrawal of estrogen at menopause appears to eliminate much of this gender difference.

There is a progressive age-related loss of orderliness of single-hormone secretion for GH, ACTH, LH, and insulin, as well as the erosion of coordinated hormone secretion for ACTH-cortisol, LH-testosterone, LH-FSH, and LH-prolactin. There are unknown mechanisms leading to age-related declines in the GH-IGF-I axis (somatopause), gonadal axis (gonadopause), and adrenal androgen secretion (adreno-pause).

New GH secretagogues, various peptidyl and non-peptidyl compounds stimulate pulsatile GH secretion and increase plasma IGF-I concentrations in adults both immediately and over intervals of days to months without producing a clinically significant down-regulation of GH responsiveness. They have a controversial value for therapeutic use in ageing men and women.

Regulation of Cognition, Body Rhythms and Sleep

Extra-glandular neurosteroids produced by CNS astroglia regulate the activity of neuronal ion-channels. The exact mechanism by which neurosteroids interact with corticosteroids to modulate the cognitive and affective changes of ageing is not known. The estrogen influences cognitive function through a feedback loop involving gonadotropin releasing hormone (GNRH), hypothalamus and neocortex and estrogen α and β receptors. In the laboratory mice, neuronal sprouting can be affected by apolipoproteins E-3 and E-4, whose production is influenced by estrogen[10]. This observation points to the presumed role of estrogen in the prevention of neuronal aging and Alzheimer's disease.

With ageing, there may come sleep fragmentation and prolonged sleep onset latency. Some GH-releasing hormones and peptides appear to trigger sleep in rats, rabbits, and humans. This normal relationship between deep sleep and GH secretion may be eroded in older adults. Sleep deprivation in young men also elicits some of the same neuroendocrine and metabolic features of ageing, such as elevated evening cortisol levels, higher sympathetic tone, and decreased glucose tolerance.

In addition, neuroendocrine rhythms are altered with ageing. The peak night-time release of melatonin decreases by approximately 50 percent with ageing. Other CNS timekeeping centers, such as the suprachiasmatic nuclei, show ageing-related alterations, as reflected in changing 24-hour rhythms of GH, prolactin, cortisol, thyroid-stimulating hormone, GH, and LH. The neuro-physiological outcomes, such as circadian and temperature rhythms, tend to show phase advance and amplitude suppression with ageing.

General Phenotype and Adult-Onset Diabetes

Body mass index (BMI) increases and visceral fat accumulates with age until early senescence. The levels of the nutritional signaling peptide leptin, mostly produced in white adipose tissue, also increase. Leptin conveys signals to the hypothalamus about fat stores and, in turn, hypothalamic efferents regulate food intake and energy expenditure. But the leptin-receptor signaling is attenuated with ageing.

About 20 percent of older adults, aged 80 or more develop type 2 diabetes mellitus. With the ageing, the insulin secretion decreases to a variable degree and becomes disorderly, resulting in a progressive increase in fasting and especially in postprandial plasma glucose levels. Simultaneously, there occurs a progressive increase in peripheral resistance to insulin action.

<u>The Ageing Adrenals and Adrenopause</u>

There is a consistent decrement in adrenal androgens (DHEA and DHEA-S) secretion with ageing both in men and women.

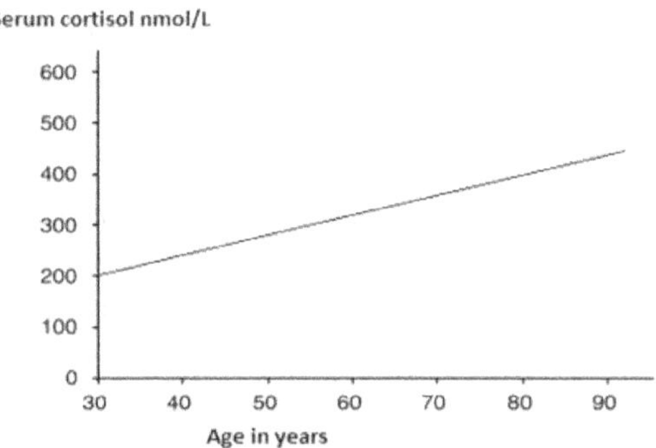

Figure 6: Cortisol secretion in ageing adults

The adrenal zona reticularis fails in ageing men and women. However, the ability of the zona fasciculata to produce cortisol is preserved (Fig 6). The receptors for mineralocorticoid and glucocorticoid in hippocampus are downregulated with age. The excessive lifelong adrenal cortisol feedback on the brain may exacerbate the ageing-associated loss in neuronal synapses and plasticity, and manifest as cognitive decline.

AGING AND GONADAL HORMONAL ALTERATIONS

The ageing is associated with significant changes in the regulation of gonadal hormonal axes and the decreased availability of their active components. The alterations occur in the functional interface between somatic physiology and gonadal endocrine systems with the ageing and result in a greater prevalence of endocrine malfunction-related disorders in the elderly population. In this context, a majority of these disorders may be potentially amenable hormonal imbalances by judicious hormonal supplementation.

The complex changes occurring in the gonadal endocrine system with ageing, have impact on the hormone production and secretion, hormone metabolism, hormone levels circulating in blood and the target tissue response to hormones. In general, the clinically identifiable changes are seen during later years of life because the physiological circadian rhythms are lost and secretion of various hormones decreases, the impact of which is augmented by the reduced sensitivity of tissues to their action.

Gonadal steroids are produced by the gonads and include estradiol and progesterone from the ovaries and testosterone from the testes. The ageing process affects the gonadal endocrine function, which have been correlated to reduced protein synthesis, a decrease in lean body mass and bone mass; increased fat mass, insulin resistance and higher cardiovascular disease risk; and fatigue, depression, anaemia, poor libido, erectile deficiency, and a decline in immune function.

There occurs prostatic enlargement in ageing men, with the gland increasing in volume and mass progressively. Albeit androgen-dependent, this propensity is also modulated by certain unknown environmental and genetic factors. Estradiol and various growth factors act locally to promote prostate epithelial and stromal growth. The contribution of sex steroids to the development and progression of the CVD is related to the clustering of interrelated risk factors that promote the development of atherosclerosis and insulin resistance[11].

The failing gonadal steroids manifest clinically as andropause in men and menopause in women (Fig 7).

MENOPAUSAL MANIFESTATIONS

Asymptomatic	Mild/Vague	Moderate	Severe
	- Mood fluctuations - Hot flushes	- Vasomotor - Uro-genital - Psychogenic	- Osteoporosis - Fracture risk

ANDROPAUSAL MANIFESTATIONS

Asymptomatic	Mild/Vague	Moderate	Severe
	- ↓ Vitality - Asthenia - Sarcopenia	- Erectile dysfunction - Unexplained depression	- PADAM - Cognitive decline

Fig 7. Clinical manifestations of menopause and andropause.

The Testosterone Story:
Andropause in Men

The testosterone has favourable direct vasodilatory effects on coronary vasculature and peripheral system vascular resistance and positive effects on cardiac and skeletal muscle function. There is testosterone-mediated control of the musculoskeletal system and age-related testosterone deficiency may result in loss of muscle mass and muscle strength, and sarcopenia. The relationship between testosterone and heart disease in both males and females is less clear. Further, the testosterone might provide metabolic benefits including improved insulin sensitivity and favourable changes in body composition. The testosterone deficiency as indicated by low serum testosterone concentrations or hypotestosteronemia, is a common hormonal alteration strongly associated with male ageing.

Testosterone is essential for the maintenance of libido and fertility, and its deficiency has been correlated to depressive symptoms with a syndrome called partial androgen deficiency of the aging male (PADAM). The andropause is a relatively ill-defined process characterised by a progressive age-dependent loss of the anabolic androgen testosterone in males[12]. The decline in testosterone levels with age, is gradual and much less dramatic than the decline of estrogens in women, and rarely affects sperm production until very old age.

The andropause is associated with a sexual dysfunction, called erectile dysfunction (ED), in the older adult male. The cognitive decline, visceral obesity, osteopenia, and relative sarcopenia also accompany androgen deficiency in ageing. Testosterone supplementation has been proved to be effective, for improving quality of life of aged patients with PADAM.

**Declining Ovarian Hormones:
Menopause in Women**

The Oestrogens act in target tissues through oestrogen receptors and G protein-coupled oestrogen receptor-1. With increasing age, the ovaries decrease in both size and weight and become progressively less sensitive to gonadotropins. There occurs a decline in the peripheral levels of oestrogen and progesterone, with an increase in luteinizing hormone (LH), follicle-stimulating hormone (FSH) and sex hormone-binding globulin. Premenopausal women have a reduced risk of CVD compared with age-matched men, but mortality as a result of CVD is higher in premenopausal women than in age-matched men. The protective role of oestrogens as relates to CVD is not fully established.

There is no biochemical signal that indicates the onset of menopause. However, serum FSH levels tend to rise in regularly menstruating late-premenopausal women. The pulsatility and the orderliness of LH release also change before menopause. Estrogen secretion around the peri-menopause becomes variable. Even in identical twin pairs, there can be a 12- to 14-year discordance in the age of menopause. Thus, reproductive ageing in women, even with identical genetic inheritance, shows variability.

The low levels of estrogens and progesterone associated with menopause have been linked to some disease states, such as osteoporosis, atherosclerosis, and dyslipidemia. This is accompanied by diverse sequelae, including an increased risk of osteoporosis, cardiovascular and cerebrovascular disease and psychogenic disturbances[13]. The incidence of breast cancer rises with age in postmenopausal women. The estrogen receptor mediates growth-factor production and possible tumor gene induction in breast cells.

The measures to attempt to ameliorate losses in oestrogen through hormone replacement therapy (HRT) is, however, controversial as it has been related to increased risks of malignancy and vascular events[14].

(SEX) HORMONE REPLACEMENT THERAPY - (S)HRT

Following menopause, approximately 90% of circulating oestrogen is lost during the fourth and fifth decade of life and the extra-glandular production of oestrogens by aromatase expression within adipose and skin becomes the predominant source of sex steroids, with additional contribution from the adrenals. As compared to the, sudden and dramatic changes seen in women, testosterone loss seen during the andropause is insidious and variable, there being no specific age at which the process starts. The global reduction in activity across the hypothalamic-pituitary-gonadal axis and reduced GnRH is the principal factor leading to gradual testicular failure. Sex hormone-binding globulin (SHBG) levels increase with ageing, manifesting the andropause as there occurs relative decrease in free testosterone than the SHBG-bound hormone.

In both men and women, the loss of sex hormones with ageing leads to alterations in body mass, musculoskeletal changes, sexual dysfunction and long-term affectations to health and certain disease-risks. There occurs decreased libido in post-menopausal women due to loss in testosterone, which in men may manifest as erectile dysfunction[15]. The most important alteration following the menopause is osteoporosis, which is driven by reductions in metabolically active trabecular bone due to uncoupling of the bone remodelling cycle secondary to oestrogen loss and leads to an increased fracture risk in older women. While men are generally protected from the effects of pathologically decreased bone mineral density by virtue of having a higher peak bone mass, though the prevalence of osteoporosis is known to increase in the ageing males. Extent of the severity guides the initiation, maintenance and monitoring (Sex)-Hormone Replacement Therapy. There have been reported both positive and negative health outcomes associated with gonadal HRTs.

The Scope of HRT

The menopause is attended by urogenital symptoms such as urinary frequency, dysuria, incontinence and vaginal atrophy. In addition, there result symptoms due to from alterations in the set point of the hypothalamus, including recurrent hot flushes following luteinizing hormone (LH) surges, and changes in serotonin levels. Despite the incapacitating symptoms affecting health and QOL in menopausal women, the HRT has been identified to be associated with an increased risk of stroke, venous thromboembolic events and pulmonary embolism in patients treated with HRT[16].

Yet, the HRT is useful for treating vasomotor, urogenital and some psychogenic symptoms related to the menopause. In addition, it decreases osteoporosis and fracture risk. But its role in the prevention or treatment of CVD is contentious. Though, the significant increase in the risk of heart disease in women undergoing the menopause, indicates a cardioprotective role for oestrogen which is lost in later age. On the flipside, there is an increased risk for breast cancer, coronary events, venous thromboembolism, gallbladder disease and ovarian cancer in women taking HRT. Further, the clinical studies favour that when indicated, HRT should be given as short-term therapy.

Risks Associated with HRT

The current evidence is contentious as to whether the testosterone replacement therapy provides a significant advantage to men with testosterone within normal parameters for their age. The loss of sex hormones may modulate cardiovascular risk through adverse alterations in lipid profile. Additionally, the falling sex hormone concentrations may lead to increased insulin resistance.

Various previous and present pharmaco-epidemiological studies do not support any causal role between testosterone replacement therapy (TRT) and adverse CV events. Yet, TRT may represent an important new strategy for improving cholesterol and insulin resistance and reducing body fat and increasing lean muscle mass. There are potential cardiovascular risks of TRT. TRT may increase the CVD risk. On the other hand, the low serum levels of endogenous testosterone are a risk factor for cardiovascular events and cognitive decline. In general, it appears that TRT does not cause marked increases in risk of cardiovascular events[17]. There might be differential effects on cardiovascular and cerebrovascular risk related to endogenous and exogenous testosterone on cardiovascular risk.

The low endogenous serum testosterone appears to be associated with higher risk of cardiovascular disease and overall mortality in older men. TRT was not associated with overall mortality, myocardial infarction, stroke, or deep venous thrombosis events. But, as inferred by a recent study, there is a potentially higher risk of cardiovascular events in men receiving testosterone, with the risk increasing early after treatment initiation and the TRT should be individualised[18].

The aggressive marketing strategy of pharmaceutical companies has resulted in this marked increase in testosterone use. There are promises for being more alert, energetic, mentally sharp and sexually functional; to combat fatigue, low sex drive, and weight gain, with the goal of regaining the vitality of their youth. The number of testosterone prescriptions issued for middle-aged or older men with either age-related or obesity-related decline in serum testosterone levels has increased even though these conditions are not approved indications for TRT[19].

CHAPTER EIGHT

THE AGEING BRAIN:
Failing Neurocognitive Functions

MANIFESTATIONS OF AGEING OF BRAIN

Among all body organs, the ageing of human brain is most incapacitating with its fallouts on quality of life, general health and psychosocial implications. There occur progressive ageing changes in the brain though at the individual level rate and types of changes are variable. The ageing of brain entails several structural, biochemical, and functional changes in the brain as well as various cognitive changes. The changes that may affect cognition and behavior occur at the molecular, intracellular, intercellular, and neuronal tissue levels. In fact, ageing is a major risk factor for the common neurodegenerative diseases, which include mild cognitive impairment (MCI), Alzheimer's disease (AD) and Parkinson's disease (PD).

Morphological Alterations

As a person gets older, changes occur in the brain. Certain parts of the brain shrink, especially those related to memory and learning, and other complex cognitive activities. The injury due to ROS at micro-level and ensuing inflammation and degeneration compromise the neuronal ability to function, affecting three important processes: communication, metabolism, and repair and regeneration. The other types of brain cells, called glial cells, which play various critical roles apart from supporting neurons also suffer changes due to ageing process. Blood circulation in the brain decreases due to multiplicity of factors, including changes in cerebral vasculature, and is a likely cause of cognitive decline. The human brain consumes about 20 percent of the body's oxygen, and the micro- and mini-vascular disturbances (mini-strokes) are common with ageing arteries and cause a cumulative and progressive damage.

The Cognitive Impairment

The cognitive abilities change as people age, their movements, and reflexes slow and the hearing and vision weaken. An important issue is how normal brain ageing transitions to pathological ageing, giving rise to neurodegenerative disorders. The toxic protein aggregates have been identified as potential contributory factors, including amyloid beta-protein in AD, tau in frontotemporal dementia, and Lewy bodies in PD. But, despite dementia and other neurodegenerative disorders associated with ageing, the advanced imaging techniques have revealed that even into late seventies, the brain is able to regenerate and produce new neurons and restructure complex neuronal circuits. Thus, a chance of regeneration and repair exists even in the aging brain.

The ageing of the brain is due to pathophysiological changes over the period of individual lifespan. In fact, it can be compared with wear and tear plus the efforts at biological level for repair and adaptation. Various insults, infective and inflammatory, lead to subcellular, cellular and tissue abnormalities resulting in neuronal adaptation, senescence and degeneration culminating into the complex phenomenon of ageing of brain. Though the aging is not genetically programmed, genes influence the ageing of brain in multiple ways (Fig 8). The CETP (cholesteryl ester transfer protein) gene is important in this matter and its I405V variant may influence general cognitive function and pathogenesis of AD. The gene expression, in turn, is influenced by factors like a healthy lifestyle, exercise, dietary and alcohol intake, and mental activity.

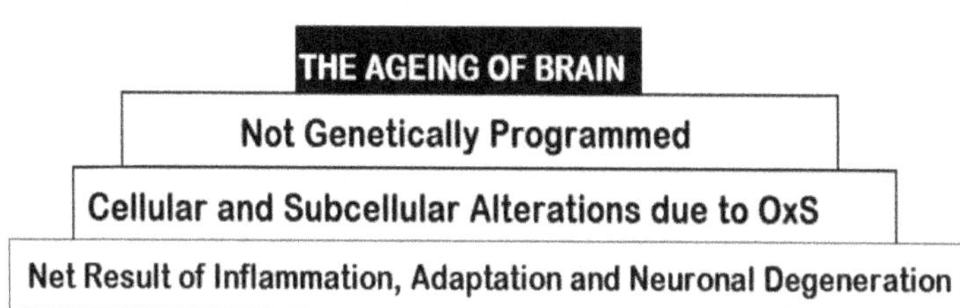

Figure 8. The factors influencing ageing of brain

The essential Cognitive Decline

With ageing, the cognitive abilities decline. On the functional level, the alterations occur due to changes in neurotransmitters and various receptors. In addition, genetics, hormones and neuroplasticity also play a role. Initially, the decline may not be apparent in form of impairment of activities of daily living (ADL), as changes are gradual and subtle. There occurs cognitive slowing, which may be evident on attentional tasks or when it is necessary to multitask or when switching from one task to another, such as driving.

Altered Information Processing: The ability to keep multiple pieces of information in mind at the same time is another skill that declines with ageing. The memory also declines, but the exact nature of the decline depends on the particular type of memory. The ability to recall new information gradually declines after 40s. The older adults are less likely than young adults to freely recall most of the new information.

Recalling a familiar name or a particular word may become tardy for older adults. The visual perceptual and scanning abilities, and spatial relationships show decline with age.

Executive functioning, such as conceptualizing a problem, making appropriate decisions, and planning and carrying out effective actions slowdown in older adults[20]. Language and vocabulary are, though, well retained throughout the lifespan.

The brain ageing interferes with performance when information is acquired in an unfamiliar situation and needs to be processed quickly. In familiar situations, older adults as compared to younger adults, tend to make more accurate interpretations of the behaviours of others when prior experience and knowledge helps to focus attention.

<u>Changes in orientation and attention</u>: The deficit in orientation is an initial and common symptoms of brain disease. The recent research suggests that normal ageing is usually not associated with significant declines in orientation, a mild deficit, though, may be a part of normal aging. In addition, many older adults suffer with a decline in attentional abilities. Since the human brain has limited attention span, people use their attention to zone in on specific stimuli and block out others. Studies have found that older adults have a more difficulty encoding and retrieving information when their attention is divided compared to younger adults. The attention may also be affected due to other factors like sensory deficits that impact older adults, for example, impaired hearing or vision.

<u>Changes in memory</u>: The memory functions, specifically those associated with the medial temporal lobe are susceptible to the age-related decline. The frontal lobes and frontal-striatal dopaminergic pathways are also affected with ageing and manifest as memory loss. With the cognitive impairment with ageing memory function is commonly affected, but there is a significant individual

variation of effects of aging on frontal lobe neurons and memory deficit.

The episodic memory and semantic memory are important with regard to ageing. Episodic memory, the information stored with tags like where, when and how, declines from middle age onwards affecting the recall in normal ageing. Semantic memory, the memory for meanings, increases gradually from middle age to the young elderly but then declines in the very elderly. These changes occur because the very elderly have slower reaction times, lower attentional levels, slower processing speeds, detriments in sensory and or perceptual functions, or potentially a lesser ability to use strategies compared to younger elderly.

<u>Changes in language</u>: With ageing, there occurs decline in the tasks related to word retrieval, comprehension of sentences, synthesis and production of sentences, affecting the totality of the verbal task. The findings from the Nun Study also underlined the linguistic decline with ageing. The increased symmetrical hemispheric activation in the frontal lobes with white matter changes is accompanied with changes in memory and language performance. Other factors such as changes in neurotransmitter or hormone levels are also important.

PHYSIOLOGICAL Vs ABNORMAL BRAIN AGEING

A number of other changes occur in the brain with ageing. The damage to white matter tracts with ageing contributes to decreased brain size and has been associated with slower information-processing and difficulty in recalling information. With ageing, the size and complexity, and the efficiency of communication between neurons become less effective and leads to various symptoms and signs of cognitive dysfunction (Fig 9). There are individual differences in ageing related cognitive decline. For some the

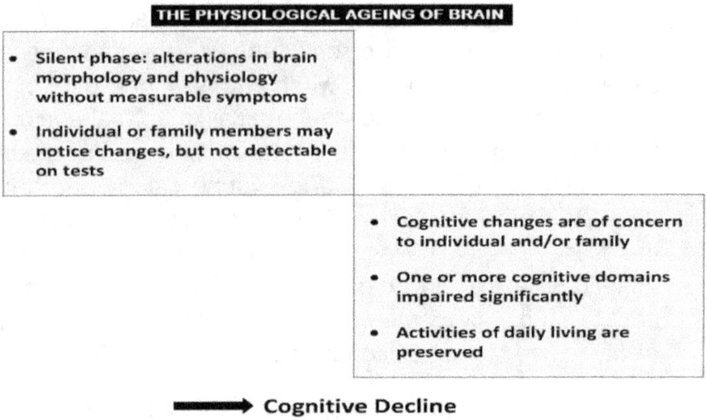

Figure 9. The physiological ageing and cognitive decline

cognitive decline with ageing is mild. It is explainable by a factor is called the cognitive reserve[21]. The level of education and lifetime of intellectual effort, which improve cognitive skills, seem to protect brain against ageing as well. The intellectual stimulus leads the brain cells to grow and regenerate, replenish loss of neurotransmitters and retards the neuronal ageing, and improves the cognitive reserve. Studies reveal that when an elderly person performs a cognitive task at the same level as that of a young adult, more brain activity is needed to maintain cognitive performance. The physical frailty with age is accompanied with proportional cognitive decline and can be levelled as normal aging process.

Both, the physiological brain ageing, and neurodegenerative disorders involve impaired energy metabolism and oxidative damage. The research indicates that mitochondria have a central role in ageing-related neurodegenerative diseases. The mitochondrial dysfunction and oxidative damage are major contributors to neuronal loss.

The neurodegenerative disease is an umbrella term for a range of conditions which primarily affect the neurons in the human brain and involve progressive loss of structure and function, leading to progressive degeneration and death of neurons, and include AD, PD, amyotrophic lateral sclerosis and Huntington's disease. The neurodegenerative process triggers neuronal cell death. Neuronal loss is a relatively late event in the neurodegenerative process, and the neuronal death is preceded by early functional alterations like electrophysiological deficits and cellular-stress-pathway activation, microanatomical deficits such as neurite retraction and synapse loss, and somal atrophy. The leading neurodegenerative disease, AD is characterized by loss of neurons and synapses in the cerebral cortex and certain subcortical areas. This loss results in gross atrophy of the affected regions, including degeneration in the temporal lobe and parietal lobe, and parts of the frontal cortex and cingulate gyrus.

The astrocytes are fundamental for homoeostasis, defense, and regeneration. There occurs loss of astroglial function and astroglial reactivity with age and contributes to the ageing of the brain as well as neurodegenerative diseases. The physiological changes in astroglia with ageing and neurodegeneration are heterogeneous.

The line of demarcation between physiological and pathological cognitive changes is not clear. The ageing is associated with several structural, biochemical, and functional alterations in the brain and these alterations may be associated several neurocognitive changes, which differ in severity. In fact, ageing is a major risk factor for the common neurodegenerative disorders, which include

MCI, AD and PD. A disproportionate cognitive decline may not be because of physiological cognitive ageing and the older adults in cognitive studies are likely to include people with undetected Alzheimer's disease (AD), cerebral vascular dementia, and other neurodegenerative diseases.

STRUCTURAL CHANGES IN AGEING BRAIN

Along with the cognitive decline. there occur changes in vasculature and white matter with ageing of brain.

<u>The cerebral volume loss</u>

There occur regional decreases in cerebral volume. But the regional volume reduction is not uniform as various tissues in the brain differ in susceptibility to age-induced changes. some brain regions shrink at a rate of up to 1% per year, whereas others remain relatively stable until late in the life. Thus, some areas such as the cingulate gyrus, and occipital cortex surrounding the calcarine sulcus are spared from the decrease in grey matter density. The proposed mechanisms of differential brain aging, include neurotransmitter systems, stress and hormonal changes, microvascular changes, calcium homeostasis, and demyelination. In general, the volume of the brain declines with age at a rate of about 5% per decade after age 40 and rate of decline increases with age over 70[22].

With the loss of cerebral volume there occurs thinning of the cortex. Most of the decrease in grey matter density occurs in dorsal, frontal, and parietal lobes on both interhemispheric and lateral brain surfaces. Ageing related loss of grey matter density in the temporal cortex appear more predominantly in the left versus right hemisphere, involving cortical language areas. These anterior language cortices have been found to mature and decline earlier than the more posterior language cortices. Further, there are sex differences in the loss of gyri and increase in sulci.

The White Matter Loss

The white matter declines with age and the myelin sheath deteriorates after around the age of 40 even in normal brain ageing. The late myelinating regions of the frontal lobes are most affected by white matter lesions. It has been suggested that there is an association between reduction in prefrontal cortical volume, increased subcortical white matter lesions, and a decreased executive function with aging.

The Changes in Neurons

The changes do not occur to the same extent in all brain regions. The temporal lobe, cerebellar vermis, cerebellar hemispheres, and hippocampus reduce in volume. The prefrontal cortex is most affected and the occipital least. Frontal and temporal lobes are most affected in men compared with the hippocampus and parietal lobes in women. The shrinking of the grey matter is frequently related to neurodegeneration or neuronal cell death.

Compared to cerebral areas, the cerebellum is protected from aging effects. With physiological brain ageing, there may occur build-up of a small neuronal protein fragment called amyloid beta. The studies suggest that amyloid plaques trigger the build-up of abnormal tau, which causes neuronal loss within brain cells in AD patients.

Neural circuits and brain plasticity

With ageing there occurs changes in the brain's ability to change structure and reassign functions leading to plasticity deficits29. It appears that the alterations in calcium regulation influence the neuronal ability to generate and propagate action potentials, which in turn affects the ability of the brain to modify its structure and reassign the functions. Further, neurotransmitters like brain-derived neurotrophic factor (BDNF) and serotonin (5-hydroxytryptamine, 5-HT) appear to play a role in neuroplasticity.

The neural circuits of some areas of brain are more vulnerable to ageing than others. Especially vulnerable neural circuits are the hippocampal and neocortical circuits. The age-related cognitive decline may in part be due to alterations at synaptic levels. The cognitive deficit also appears to be due to physiological and biochemical factors such as changes in enzymatic activity, chemical messengers, or gene expression in cortical circuits.

<u>Neurofibrillary tangles</u>

An important difference between normal brain aging and pathological changes, is the presence and distribution of neurofibrillary tangles. The neurofibrillary tangles are composed of paired helical filaments. In normal, non-pathological ageing, the number of tangles in the affected tissues is relatively low and restricted to the olfactory nucleus, para-hippocampal gyrus, amygdala and entorhinal cortex. With normal ageing, there is a small but general increase in the density of tangles. Whereas, in the pathological brain ageing, representing the neurodegenerative entity, neurofibrillary tangles are commonly found with amyloid plaques in AD patients.

<u>The Hormonal Influence</u>

Another factor to consider with regard to the ageing brain, its plasticity and cognitive performance is the hormonal influence (Fig 10). The changes in sex hormones occur with ageing, in women at menopause in and in men at andropause. Women also have higher prevalence of failing memory and a higher incidence of AD. It has been noted that it may improve with estrogen therapy which increases dopaminergic responsivity and may be protective in AD[23].

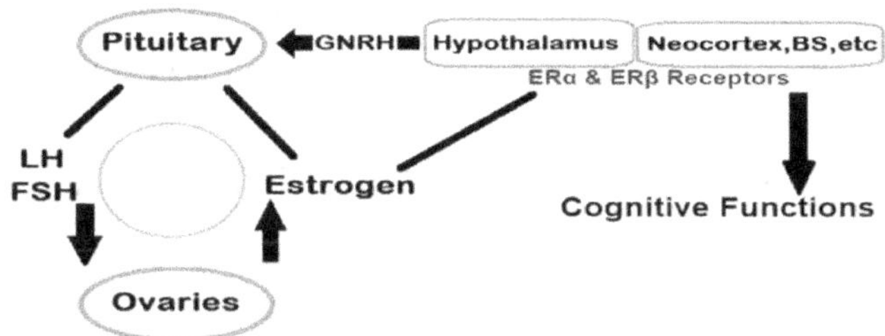

Figure 10: Hypothalamus, neocortex, GNRH and estrogen feedback loop influencing cognitive function.

Growth hormone levels also decline with age and its supplementation appears to be associated with improvement in cognitive function.

ETIOLOGICAL FACTORS FOR AGEING BRAIN

1. The cognitive decline has been attributed to oxidative stress, cytokines, inflammatory reactions and neuronal degeneration, and changes in the cerebral microvasculature (Fig 11).

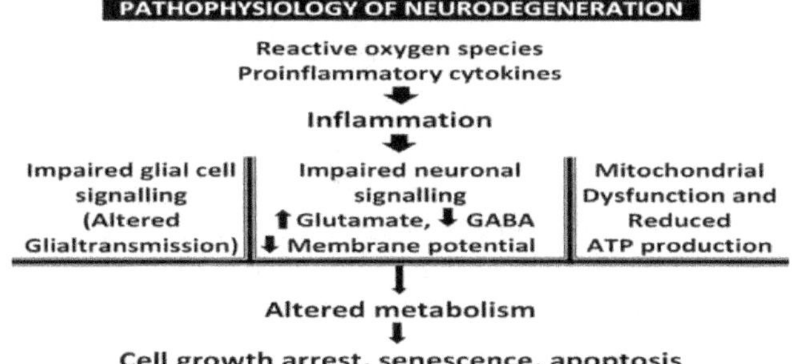

Figure 11: Theories and concepts of neurodegeneration

The difference in oxidative damage related to various lifestyle factors has been associated with individual differences in cognition impairment in healthy elderly people from mild cognitive impairment to severe decline and predisposition to neurodegenerative disorders.

2. The Genetic Factors: The variation in the effects of ageing among individuals can be attributed to both genetic and epigenetic factors. With ageing, the brain shows a decline in cognitive function and alterations in gene expression. This modulation in gene expression may be due to oxidative DNA damage at promoter regions in the genome.

The DNA damage increasingly accumulates with age in the brain and includes the oxidized nucleoside 8-hydroxy-deoxy-guanosine (8-OHdG), single- and double-strand breaks, DNA-protein crosslinks and malondialdehyde (MDA) adducts. The mitochondrial changes with ageing also affect neurons.

There are certain genes that are down-regulated over the age of 40 and include GluR1 AMPA receptor subunit, NMDA R2A receptor subunit (involved in learning), subunits of the GABA-A receptor, calmodulin 1 and CAM kinase II alpha (genes involved in long-term potentiation), and calcium signaling genes, synaptic plasticity genes, synaptic vesicle release and recycling genes. Whereas, certain genes which are upregulated include the genes associated with stress response and DNA repair. The DNA damage may reduce the expression of selectively vulnerable genes involved in learning, memory and neuronal survival, initiating a pattern of brain aging that starts early in life.

3. Neurosignaling and Neurotransmitters: In the brain, the neurotransmitters regulate each other's action and

release. A mild imbalance in the mutual regulation has been linked to temperament variations in healthy people. Whereas the severe imbalances or disruptions in neurotransmitter systems have been associated with disorders like depression, insomnia, attention deficit hyperactivity disorder (ADHD), anxiety, memory loss, Parkinson's disease etc. The chronic stress can be a contributor to neurotransmitter system changes. The genetics also plays a role in neurotransmitter activities.

A neuron transports information by a nerve impulse called the action potential. When an action potential arrives at the synapse's presynaptic terminal button, it may stimulate release of neurotransmitters. These neurotransmitters are released into the synaptic cleft to bind onto the receptors of the postsynaptic membrane and influence another neuron, either in an inhibitory or excitatory way, with the probability that it will induce an action potential. Each neuron receives a multitude of excitatory and inhibitory signals every second. The type I (excitatory) synapses are typically located on the shafts or the spines of dendrites, whereas type II (inhibitory) synapses are typically located on a cell body.

The ageing process entails various biochemical changes in brain. A number of neurotransmitters, as well as their receptors exhibit alterations in various regions of the brain with the ageing process. The major neurotransmitter systems include the noradrenaline (norepinephrine) system, the dopamine system, the serotonin system, and the cholinergic system, and the trace amines, which have a very significant effect on neurotransmission in monoamine pathways (i.e., dopamine, histamine, norepinephrine, and serotonin pathways) throughout the brain. The most prevalent transmitter in human brain is glutamate, which is excitatory at over 90% of the synapses. The next most prevalent neurotransmitter is

Gamma-Aminobutyric Acid, or GABA, which is inhibitory at more than 90% of the synapses that do not use glutamate. In addition, there are over 50 neuroactive peptides e.g. β-endorphin. Certain other transmitters are used in fewer synapses, albeit they are important.

The neurotransmitters most important with regard to ageing are dopamine and serotonin. The serotonin and BDNF levels also fall with ageing. Another factor, monoamine oxidase, increases with age and may be responsible for excess liberation of free radicals that exceed the inherent antioxidant reserves.

The dopaminergic pathways regulate cognitive processes and behaviours such as arousal (wakefulness), aversion, cognitive control and working memory (co-regulated by norepinephrine), emotion and mood, motivation, motor function, positive reinforcement, reward (primary mediator), sexual arousal, orgasm, and refractory period (via neuroendocrine regulation). The dopamine functions in the brain include regulation of motor behavior, pleasures related to motivation and emotional arousal. It also plays a critical role in the reward system. Parkinson's disease has been linked to low levels of dopamine and schizophrenia has been linked to high levels of dopamine.

There occur age-related changes in brain in dopamine synthesis, and its binding and receptors. Also, there is a significant age-related decrease in D1, D2 and D3 dopamine receptors. The dopaminergic pathways between the frontal cortex and the striatum decline with increasing age, levels of dopamine decline, and synapses/receptors are reduced or binding to receptors is reduced. In fact, there occurs a general decrease in D-receptor density with age and a significant age-related decline in dopamine receptors in the anterior cingulate cortex, frontal cortex, lateral temporal cortex, hippocampus, medial temporal cortex, amygdala, medial thalamus, and lateral thalamus. The dopamine deficiency with age is responsible for associated with declines in cognitive and motor performance and various neurological symptoms that increase in frequency with age, such as decreased arm swing and increased rigidity, and age-related changes in cognitive flexibility.

The serotonergic pathways regulate cognitive processes and behaviours such as arousal (wakefulness), body temperature regulation, emotion, and mood, potentially including aggression, feeding and energy homeostasis, sensory perception and have a minor role in reward response. Serotonin influences appetite, sleep, memory and learning, temperature, mood, behavior, muscle contraction, and function of the cardiovascular system and endocrine system. Decrease in serotonin receptors and the serotonin transporter occurs with age. With age the number of the S1 receptors in the caudate nucleus, putamen, and frontal cerebral cortex decrease. There is also a decreased binding capacity for serotonin transporter in the thalamus and midbrain.

Glutamate is another important neurotransmitter that tends to decrease with age. There occurs a significant decline with age, especially in parietal gray matter, basal ganglia, and frontal white matter. The parietal and basal ganglia regions are often affected in degenerative brain diseases and show decreased glutamate concentration and activity.

4. Vascular factors: The white matter lesions (WML) have been related to increased cerebrovascular risk and a reduction in cerebral blood flow, cerebral reactivity and vascular density. They may also be associated with further tissue changes in grey matter. The WML are found more in frontal rather than posterior brain regions. They seem to impair frontal lobe function regardless of their location. Further, the WML increase with age and show levels of heritability and are common in the elderly even when asymptomatic. Associated with ageing and related to blood pressure and vascular factors, other changes

include strokes and small vessel disease. The research provides evidence that vascular factors contribute to cognitive dysfunction with ageing.

Further, the vascular dementia (VaD) is most frequent in the elderly amounting to about 15%–30%, second only to AD, which is found in about 40%–70% cases[24]. Risk factors to ageing and development of VaD include hypertension, diabetes, hyperhomocysteinaemia, and a high cholesterol. The prevalence of dementia increases almost exponentially with increasing age with around 20% of those aged 80 affected rising to 40% of those aged 90[25].

5. Hormonal factors: The deranged thyroid function bears a relationship cognitive function[26]. Hypothyroidism as well as hyperthyroidism are associated with cognitive decline (Fig 12).

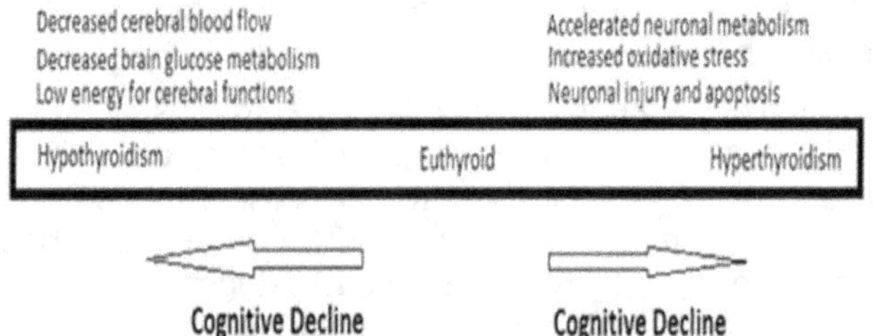

Figure 12: Hypothyroidism and hyperthyroidism are associated with cognitive decline

The failing sex hormones in men with andropause and in women at menopause, and fall in growth hormone in both, affect cognitive function with ageing. The research suggests that estrogen therapy in women may increase dopaminergic responsivity. The hormone replacement therapy (HRT) appears to play a protective role.

CHAPTER NINE

THE AGEING HEART:
Enduring Cardiovascular deficit

AGEING AND CV DISORDERS

Age is the most important determinant of cardiovascular (CV) health. There occur pathophysiological alterations at macro level including altered ventricular systolic and diastolic functions and diminished cardiac reserve, cardiac hypertrophy, increased arterial stiffness, and impaired endothelial function. Simultaneously, important changes are taking place at micro level; at cellular, subcellular and molecular levels. In this perspective, there occurs a progressive but varying decline in CV physiological functions and an exponential rise in both the CV risk and incidence and prevalence of atherosclerosis, hypertension, coronary artery disease (CAD) or coronary heart disease (CHD) and heart failure (HF), cerebrovascular and peripheral vascular disease in older adults parallel with the advancing age.

Statistically, the older adults (>60 years old) account for more than 80% of coronary heart disease, more than 75% of congestive HF, and more than 70% of atrial fibrillation (AF) patients[27]. It is estimated that by 2030, approximately 20% of the population will be aged 65 or older, and in this age group, CVDs will amount to over 40% of all deaths and rank as the leading cause of disability and suboptimal quality of life during later years[28,29].

To prove this point, various studies including the Framingham Heart Study and the Baltimore Longitudinal Study on Ageing highlight the changes that occurs with age in healthy humans, and their association and relevance to the increased incidence of left ventricular hypertrophy (LVH), chronic HF, and AF seen with advancing age[30]. With aging, the declining cardioprotective systems and increasing disease processes predispose to the development of HF, which is largely a disease of the elderly. About 50% of all HF diagnoses and 90% of all HF deaths occur in this segment of the population[31].

AGEING AND CV ALTERATIONS

In apparently normal ageing healthy individuals, from the age of 20 to 85 years, there is a gradual increase in Left ventricle (LV) wall thickness, alterations in the diastolic filling pattern, impaired LV ejection and HR reserve capacity, and altered heart rhythm. The age-associated increase in arterial stiffness contributes at least partly to cause the age-associated increase in blood pressure. These age-associated changes compromise the cardiac reserve capacity and affect the threshold for symptoms and signs. There occurs a progressive decline in LV compliance with age, which may go unnoticed and manifest in stressful situations. The HF, in the older adults, is often a consequence of age-related alterations in blood pressure and cardiac and vascular structure and function.

<u>Arterial Stiffening</u>: There occurs an age-associated increase in intimal media (IM) thickening and a reduction in compliance signifying an increase in arterial stiffness. The arterial stiffness influences the development of atherosclerosis, which through endothelial cell dysfunction and other mechanisms, promotes vascular stiffness. Various risk factors, including hypertension, smoking, dyslipidemia, diabetes, diet, and certain undefined genetic factors, interact with vascular ageing to activate an atherosclerotic plaque formation. The atherosclerosis,

thus, increases with ageing due to an interaction of vascular ageing with various atherosclerotic risk factors.

<u>Altered arterial Pressure</u>: The elevated pulse pressure is an independent risk factor for future CV events and studies have shown that individuals manifesting elevations in systolic and pulse pressures are more likely to develop clinical disease. The age-dependent increase in blood pressure contributes to LVH, which is an independent risk factor for CVD. There occurs an age-dependent rise in average systolic blood pressure across all adult age groups, whereas the average diastolic pressure rises until 50 years of age, levels off from ages 50 to 60, and declines thereafter. Owing to the decline in diastolic pressure and rise in systolic pressure, isolated systolic hypertension is the most common form of hypertension in older adults associated with an increased risk for CVD.

<u>LV Afterload and Vascular Afterload</u>: The optimal ejection fraction occurs when ventricular and vascular loads are matched. The precise cardiac and vascular load matching in younger persons is preserved in older adults at rest. However, during exercise a mismatch occurs due to altered LV and vascular elastance and responsible for the deficit in the LV ejection fraction (EF) reserve.

<u>Heart Rhythm (HR)</u>: The HR variability declines steadily with age and has been linked to increased risk for CV morbidity and mortality. There is an increase in the prevalence and complexity of both supraventricular and ventricular arrhythmias at rest, ambulatory, or during exercise in otherwise healthy older adults. AF is detected in approximately 3% to 4% of healthy volunteers over age 60 years, which is 10-fold higher than in the general adult population.

85

<u>Age-dependent LV Changes</u>: Based on data from Framingham Heart Study and Baltimore Longitudinal Study on Ageing, from apparently healthy adults, there occurs an age-dependent increase in LV wall thickness measured by echocardiography in both men and women, indicating increased prevalence of LVH with age, even in the absence of clinical hypertension. The LVH is associated with increased risk for CHD, sudden death, stroke, and overall CVD burden.

Left ventricular diastolic dysfunction is highly prevalent in older adults, and adversely affects the exercise capacity and predisposes to the development of diastolic heart failure. The LVEF is preserved during aging, though the maximum EF achievable during exercise, decreases with age. The value of EF less than 50% is indicative of impaired LV systolic function.

<u>Aortic and Mitral Valvular changes</u>: With ageing, there occurs myxomatous degeneration and collagen deposition leading to valvular sclerosis. Aortic valve sclerosis is present in 30%–80% of older adults, and often develops in parallel with progression of atherosclerosis in other vessels and accompanied by an increased occurrence of CV events and mortality. The valvular changes superimposed on ventricular changes in older adults result in a severe compromise in the cardiac functional reserve capacity, make the heart more susceptible to stress and lower the threshold for disease-related symptoms and signs.

<u>Altered Neurohormonal Regulation</u>: The renin-angiotensin aldosterone system (RAAS) is the key neurohormonal system that regulates blood pressure and stress induced response. The RAAS has been linked to age-related declines in cardiac function. The intracardiac concentrations of angiotensin (Ang) II, the main effector

hormone is increased with age, and responsible for various CV structural, functional, and molecular changes.

With ageing, there is apparent deficits in sympathetic modulation due to altered B-adrenergic signalling, which modulates HR and contractility and redistributes blood to body systems. With age, there occur increased plasma levels of norepinephrine and epinephrine due to an increased spill-over into the circulation, and a reduced plasma clearance due to decreased norepinephrine re-uptake at nerve endings. The deficient sympathetic modulatory component leads to deficient CV regulation including HR and filling time, afterload - both cardiac and vascular, and myocardial contractility.

There is an age-related alteration in natriuretic peptides signalling. The plasma levels of both, atrial natriuretic peptide (ANP) and brain natriuretic peptide (BNP) increase with age in populations without CVD. There is an increased secretion of BNP by ventricular cardiomyocytes in setting of volume or pressure overload and ischemia, and in response to various neuroendocrine stimuli including endothelin I and Ang II.

PATHOPHYSIOLOGY OF CV ALTERATIONS

The ageing is an independent risk factor for atherosclerosis, as the vascular cellular senescence contributes to atherosclerosis.

<u>Cardiac Aging, Cardiomyopathy and HF</u>: In a response to increased vascular resistance, there occurs remodelling of myocardium which includes myocyte hypertrophy and alterations in extracellular matrix (ECM). The cardiac hypertrophy results in increased myocardial oxygen demand and decreased coronary perfusion pressure due to compression of the coronary microcirculation. This

causes mismatch in oxygen/nutrient supply-demand and induces a relative myocardial ischemia. At the subcellular level, mitochondrial oxidative stress and dysfunction play an important role in cardiac ageing (Fig 13).

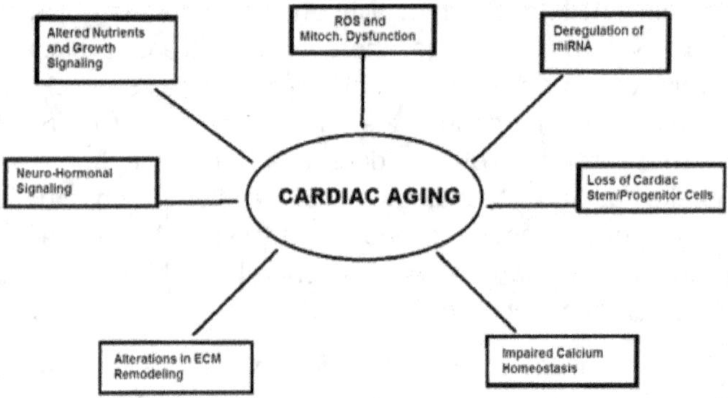

Figure 13: The molecular mechanisms of cardiac ageing

These changes reduce functional reserve and predispose the aged hearts to the development of HF. The HF adversely affects the cardiac pumping capacity, and in most cases is asymptomatic for a variable period. The symptomatic HF patients represent the visible part of an iceberg and best defined as the acute decompensation of chronic HF (Fig 14). There is a rising incidence of HF worldwide and it is a major health concern carrying an increased morbidity and potential loss of work days, hospitalization and substantial cost of treatment. Furthermore, its clinical course is gradually progressive, which affects quality of life (QOL) especially during later years of life.

At the cellular and subcellular levels, the HF is associated with defects in mitochondrial function. The alterations in substrate metabolism contribute to contractile dysfunction and LV remodeling. In the advanced stages of HF, the myocardium has low ATP content due to a decreased ability to generate ATP by oxidative metabolism and loss of contractile strength.

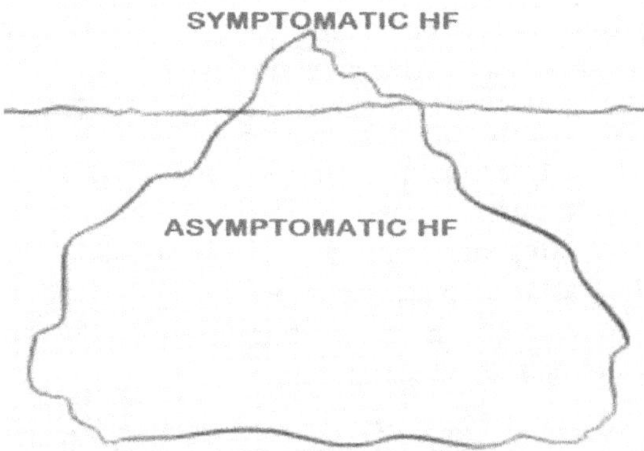

Figure 14: The Concept of HF Iceberg

There is a progressively reduced myocardial performance, due to the loss of myocardial tissue and dysfunctional viable myocytes. Myocardial metabolism is altered and the substrate utilization switches from mostly fatty acids to glucose. In addition to metabolic derangements, there is increased adrenergic tone which adds further to metabolic dysregulation and the progression of myocardial dysfunction.

Reactive Oxygen Species and Oxidative Stress: The incidence of CVDs correlates with age, which in turn appears to be the result of oxidative stress and cumulative damage at cellular and molecular levels. At a cellular level, the oxidative damage to mitochondria results in acidification of the cytoplasm and release of cytochrome c. At the subcellular level there is damage to DNA and other subcellular structures, and gradual loss of the telomere cap, due to several reactive molecular species that include reactive oxygen species (ROS) and reactive nitrogen species, reactive aldehyde species, transition metal intermediates and advanced glycation end (AGE) products. The oxidative stress leading to irreversible damage signals either cell cycle arrest or apoptosis heralding the aging process at the tissue level.

There occurs an age-dependent alteration in mitochondrial oxidative phosphorylation function, which is related to impaired electron transport function and increased electron leakage and generation of mitochondrial ROS. As an organ with a high metabolic demand and rich in mitochondria, the heart is particularly vulnerable to mitochondrial oxidative damage.

Mitochondrial Oxidative Stress and Cardiac Ageing: The ROS production increases with age and the cardiomyocytes become more susceptible to oxidative stress and undergo apoptosis and necrosis. The necrosis promotes in proinflammatory and profibrotic environment. The rate of cardiomyocytes regeneration from cardiac stem cells pool is inadequate to maintain cardiomyocyte numbers to replenish cardiomyocyte loss, resulting cardiac senescence and proneness to HF.

There occurs deterioration in mitochondrial energetics with HF. The studies in mice have documented an age-dependent increase in mitochondrial protein-carbonylation, which is indicative of increased oxidative damage to mitochondrial proteins. The accumulation of mitochondrial DNA mutations increases apoptosis and leads to development of cardiomyopathy with marked LVH, systolic and diastolic dysfunction, and an overall impaired myocardial performance.

Neurohormonal Accompaniments of Cardiac Oxidative Stress: As mentioned earlier, the RAAS has been linked to CVD and age-related decline in cardiac function. The increased intracardiac Ang II concentrations with age, induces an increase in total cellular and mitochondrial ROS, oxidative stress and consequent myocardial damage. The inhibition of Ang II signaling by an angiotensin converting enzyme inhibitor enalapril or angiotensin receptor type I inhibitor losartan, in animal experiments, have been shown to slow down the onset of age-related CV pathologies. These drugs also reduced myocardial fibrosis and fibrosis-related arrhythmias in aged mice[32,33].

The acute β-adrenergic stimulation induces a cAMP and protein kinase A(PKA)-dependent increase in mitochondrial ROS in ventricular cardiomyocytes. Experimentally, the chronic βadrenergic stimulation induces mitochondrial membrane depolarization and cardiomyocyte apoptosis in adult mice. Further, the adenylyl cyclase type 5 (AC5) disruption, which is involved in β-adrenergic downstream signalling, protected mice against age-dependent cardiac hypertrophy, systolic dysfunction, apoptosis, and fibrosis and lead to an increased lifespan. In clinical trials, the beta-blockers (β-adrenergic receptor inhibitors) have demonstrated a clear benefit for survival in patients with heart failure[34].

Atrial natriuretic peptide (ANP) and brain natriuretic peptide (BNP) bind to membrane-bound guanylase cyclase receptors to exert the physiological effect for maintaining hemodynamics through body fluid and electrolyte homeostasis. The plasma levels of both of them increase with age. In clinical studies, human ANP (carperitide) has been shown to suppress thioredoxin, reduce oxidative stress, and improve the symptoms and hemodynamics of patients with HF. Whereas another peptide, C-natriuretic peptide (CNP) has an antiproliferative effect and is reciprocally associated with LV fibrosis, and progressively declines with age.

<u>Vascular Cell Senescence in Diabetic Patients</u>: Insulin resistance and hyperinsulinemia are essential features of T2DM. The findings suggest that diabetes promotes the senescence of endothelial cells via the insulin/Akt pathway and/or the high glucose–induced signaling pathway, resulting in the development of diabetic vascular complications. The increased plasma and tissue levels of proinflammatory cytokines and prothrombogenic factors exacerbate insulin resistance and to contribute to diabetic complications.

CELLULAR AND SUBCELLULAR CHANGES IN CV DISEASE

<u>The Concept of Genome Stability and Ageing</u>: The age-dependent changes occur in both the heart and vasculature, which undergo numerous alterations at cellular and subcellular levels as a result of deregulation of various molecular longevity pathways. A number of diverse stimuli induce senescence. But they appear to converge on certain pathways that influence cell cycle regulation, DNA repair and apoptosis, and the process of cellular senescence (Fig 15).

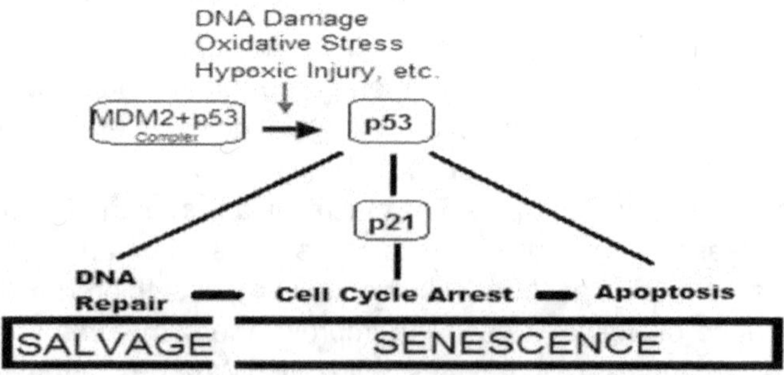

Figure 15: The Concept of Genome Stability and Ageing

These pathways are regulated by the tumor suppressor proteins p53 and pRb. The p53 is a crucial mediator of the cellular response to damaged DNA and dysfunctional telomeres, and in turn activates the cyclin-dependent inhibitor p21. It is considered that senescence occurs via the p53 pathway in response to DNA damage and telomere dysfunction[35].

<u>Angiogenesis and Vascular Ageing</u>: Angiogenesis, another critical mechanism, is responsible for repairing tissues after damage caused by daily wear and tear and events such as myocardial ischemia and infarction and cerebrovascular stroke[36].

The age-related impairment of angiogenesis contributes to end-organ damage and affects cardiovascular health. Processes and pathways contributing to impairment of angiogenesis, include cellular senescence, telomere attrition, oxidative damage, NO, hypoxia, and vascular growth factors.

CHAPTER TEN
SECRETS TO LONGEVITY:
Theories of Ageing

THE GENETIC KEY
FOR LONGEVITY

All life forms age. In fact, Ageing is a fact of life. It has been an enigma for generations. But now the molecular biologists experimenting with organisms such as yeast, roundworms, fruit flies, and mice have succeeded in increasing the life span by altering single genes. The experimentally altered organisms tend to live longer and age more slowly. Further, it seems that the genetic manipulations causing these changes work through certain common pathways across various species. Thus, there seems to be an evolutionary biological program that modulates and controls ageing.

The Worm-side Story:

The tiny roundworms, Caenorhabditis elegans, when exposed to environmental stress during their development, enter into a state akin to hibernation by modifying themselves into a spore like forms, called dauers. They can remain in the suspended condition for long periods, till the surroundings again become hospitable to growth. This phenomenon is an indication that organisms can, as part of physiology, regulate their life span. This also means that genes control longevity. It was demonstrated later on that the roundworms missing one copy of a gene called daf-2 during development could enter the dauer state regardless of environmental conditions.

By altering the single gene - called daf-2 in the DNA, scientists could double the lifespan of C. elegans. The daf-2 appears to be a master control gene, and by altering it, functions of various other genes in the worm's DNA can be modified. These other genes do functions, such as, making antioxidant proteins that protect the cells from oxidative damage, protecting the cells from bacterial infections, etc. Thus, as consequence of altering a single gene, it was possible to significantly enhance lifespan in C. elegans[37].

Mitochondrial gene mutations:

The genetic mutations in mitochondria appear to trigger changes leading the cells to die and speed up the ageing process. By altering a gene called polymerase gamma, which functions as a spellchecker during the copying of mitochondrial DNA in mice led them to age fast[38]. Around eight or nine months of age there were having plenty of signs of ageing, such as greying of hair, loss of bone mass, loss of muscle mass, and defects in the spinal curvature.

Because the mitochondria also control the natural process of cell death, called apoptosis, mistakes by the spell-checking gene can cause cells to die. As mitochondrial mutations accumulate, there are increased cell deaths and appearance of the ageing characteristics. This phenomenon may be linked to ageing in humans.

There are certain mechanisms through which the body controls mitochondrial mutations and inhibits cell death. The studies indicate existence of a set of genes, which function to prolong life and to inhibit the effects of mitochondrial mutations.

The Predictors of Longevity

The early circumstances of human life, such as the month of birth, may have a profound effect later on the survival and ageing[39]. The critical periods early in early childhood may involve seasonal variations in living conditions, availability of nutrients and exposure to pathogens.

The studies also show that paternal age at person's conception may be an important predictor of lifespan[40]. This may be related to the mutation load or other genetic damage in maternal ovum or paternal sperm cells playing a significant role in determining the human lifespan.

Further, there is an unusual pattern of human lifespan inheritance. It has been discovered that there is no lifespan heritability if parental lifespan is below a threshold age of 75-85 years but there is a strong heritability of lifespan if parents have lived longer[41].

Other multiple factors:

When the researchers altered daf-2 as well as reproductive hormones, the worms lived six times as long as normal and stayed young and healthy[42]. They looked disease-resistant and did not get age-related diseases until they were much older than normal. These experiments indicate that ageing is under genetic control, rather than just a consequence of wear and tear.

It has been discovered that genes daf-2 and age-1 (another gene), are part of the same molecular pathway. In fact, there are not many genes in the pathway that regulate ageing. The finding that daf-2 also encodes an insulin receptor, has linked ageing to another program that can extend life span in any organism, namely, the caloric restriction (CR).

DIET AND CALORIC RESTRICTION

The Caloric Restriction

In the 1930's, the researchers discovered that they could extend the life of rats by 33 percent if they put them on a very low-calorie diet[43]. These animals lived longer, suffered fewer late-life diseases, appeared more youthful, and their biological ageing was slowed. Similar life-extending studies have been reported in other organisms, ranging from fruit flies to fish. In general, the CR regimen protects against disease and slows ageing (Fig 16). The animals on CR have lower levels of circulating blood glucose, insulin, and triglycerides.

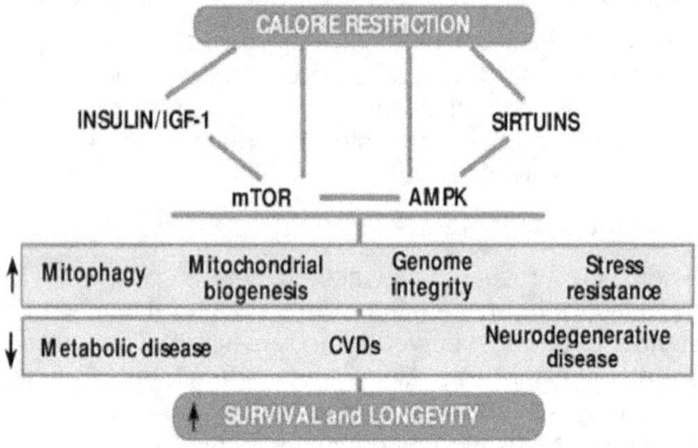

Figure 16: Pathways linking CR to health and longevity

In this context, limiting fat, protein or carbohydrate, without accompanying caloric reduction, does not increase the maximum lifespan. The supplementation with extra antioxidants and multivitamins also does not increase lifespan. Varying the types of fats, carbohydrates and proteins ingested also does not have any effect. In fact, no other intervention except caloric restriction has yet been shown to slow ageing.

It seems probable that caloric restriction is an effective way to prolong life. The low-calorie intake may work by reducing the amount of free radical produced. There are less mitochondrial mutations and less programmed cell deaths. The effects of CR on lifespan, disease and ageing processes are applicable to virtually all species.

But CR is not without certain adverse effects. There occur hunger pangs, a decreased ability to handle stresses, such as cold temperatures or infection, loss of libido and infertility, osteoporosis, and loss of muscle mass. The caloric restriction is not easy to practise. People under 20 are advised against caloric restricted diets.

Sparse Diets and Lower Body weight for Longer Life

Reducing consumption of dietary calories is the only intervention of proven value in extending the average and maximum lifespan. The data indicate that more the caloric restriction, more is the potential life extension - a pattern that holds good until caloric restriction becomes actual starvation, whereupon it shortens lifespan. The adult-onset caloric restriction should be phased in gradually to allow appetite to adjust and accompanied by a nutrient-enriched diet.

The Japanese district of Okinawa has the longest average lifespan in the world and the highest percentage of centenarians - people living to 100 or more. The Okinawans eat up to 40 percent fewer calories than Americans and about 20 percent fewer calories than the Japanese average. But their diet has adequate essential ingredients. The result, thus, Okinawans have a reduced mortality and enjoy reduced morbidity from a number of diseases.

An optimal CR reduces the incidence of virtually all diseases of ageing such as cancer, heart disease, diabetes, osteoporosis, auto-immune disorders, neurological decline and diseases such as Alzheimer's and Parkinson's diseases. Eating less is associated with lower weight, which in turn is associated with longer life as shown by studies in centenarians.

The Dietary Choices and Health and Longevity

A diet is essentially a lifestyle choice. It may change over time because of the availability of food or with change in preference. One may alter one's diet in the light of new knowledge. A healthy diet is generally expected to incorporate a wide variety of foods. But there is no single best diet for everyone. There is enormous phenotypic variation among human beings (e.g. height, bone density, skin-fold thickness, body fat, fat-free mass, and body fat distribution). This variation is responsible for varying micro- and macro-nutrient requirements.

In addition, there is a considerable variation in dietary needs at different exercise levels and at different age groups. Added to this, is the issue of an immediate gratification (like taste, indulgence, luxurious eating, etc.) Versus deferred substantial gains (increased lifespan, youthfulness and freedom from many diseases) later.

The Dietary Composition and Controversies

The average diet has about 35 percent fat (12% saturated, 3% trans-fats, 14% monounsaturated, and 6% polyunsaturated), 50 percent carbohydrate, and 15 percent protein. The diet advisory recommends a change from this eating pattern. Whereas some believe in very high carbohydrate and very low-fat diets (notably, Ornish regimen); others believe in moderately high protein and very high fat and very low carbohydrates (Atkins' regimen); still others recommend higher protein, less saturated fat, but more polyunsaturated and monounsaturated fats (Sears' regimen), and more mono and poly fats, with reduced carbohydrates (Reaven's regimen).

<u>Dietary Composition: Macro-nutrients</u>

The modern diet may look like the recommended diet but has more saturated fat and a bit less carbohydrate. The heart disease is related to saturated fat. The extra weight due to too much food can cause abnormal carbohydrate metabolism and lead to development of diabetes. Further, the carbohydrates consumed in the actual modern diet are low in nutrients (potatoes, breads, etc.) and often lead to 'crowding out' of vegetables and fruits.

The consensus is that CR increases the need for protein intake, relative to non-caloric restricted diets. The protein intake should be doubled from 0.8 gm/kg of body weight/day to 1.6g/kg/day. By substantially curtailing starches and sugars, one can increase the proportion of the nutritionally dense, but low-calorie vegetables and fruits.

<u>The Carbohydrates and Glycemic Index</u>

The glucose-insulin metabolic loop is a feedback control. When we eat high glycemic index carbohydrates and, thus, putting more total glucose into our system, some of this glucose forms cross-links with proteins, called non-enzymatic glycosylation. These cross-links enhance ageing. In addition, the raised glucose after a meal leads to increased insulin in the bloodstream, required to enable glucose to go into the cells. More insulin helps temporarily but promotes insulin resistance and metabolic syndrome. Because of these two reasons, a low-glycemic index food is to be preferred.

Thus, fasting on certain days (getting the same number of calories by alternating days with no food with days with lots of food) or erratic intake of food during the day (missing a meal followed by a heavy meal) is likely to result in greater fluctuations of insulin, than eating more evenly. An essentially continuous nutrient flow is considered the best way to even blood glucose and minimize insulin output. Also, caloric restriction may become more difficult with practice of fasting on certain days.

Mechanism of CR
CR in Action

The CR extends maximum and average life spans and improves disease resistance, including resistance to many cancers. It probably does this by a reduction in the accumulation of oxidant and free-radical damage, or because ingestion of fewer calories favourably alters fat deposition, obesity, and hormones. There takes place an improvement in the immune response, as well.

When practicing CR, one has to reduce everything in proportion. Thus, the calorie intake is reduced but the ratio of protein, carbohydrates, and fats is maintained on lines of a balanced diet.

It can be done by:

- Curtailing the 'whites' (bread, potatoes, pasta, and rice) - They have poor nutrition value and a high glycemic index, resulting in excessive insulin production and insulin resistance.
- Curtailing the desserts and the snacks for the similar reason. Taking fruits to substitute for the desserts. Substituting drinks like juices, tea and coffee for low-calorie or empty-calorie drinks.
- Curtailing saturated fats: Reducing visible fat and substitute liquid oils for butter, use toned instead of full fat milk.
- Eating more vegetables of all kinds. Increasing fish consumption, especially high omega-3 oil varieties.

The CR and
Role of Exercise

The exercise helps, both physically and mentally. There occur a number of molecular changes in the brain during exercise. It increases the production of brain-derived neurotrophic factor (BDNF), which protects nerve cells and increases the number of nerve cells that are involved in various aspects of memory and cognition.

The human brain begins to shrink in volume at about age 30, and as a normal process of ageing continues to lose volume until the end of life. Various studies indicate that the aerobic exercise slows down the loss of brain tissue in older adults. These effects are predominantly seen in three key areas of the brain: the frontal, temporal and parietal regions. The frontal region regulates memory, planning, scheduling, decision-making, etc. The temporal region is related to memory and memory consolidation. The parietal region is related to recall and navigation.

It may appear strange, but losing weight via increased caloric expenditure, i.e. exercise, does not give CR's health benefits. The reason lies in the free radical concept. The food is the source of 90 percent of the oxidants or free radicals. Reducing food intake will reduce oxidative damage. Exercise, in fact, contributes to increased free radical generation by burning food faster. But these negative effects are more than offset by health benefits of exercise, so the average lifespan is certainly increased by exercise.

As such, the exercise may not add anything to the maximum lifespan and fairly little to the average lifespan when there is already a calorie restriction.

Stabilizing Proteins:
The Sirtuins

The yeast is a single-celled fungus whose life span is defined by the number of times it can divide. It divides 20 times on average—40 times at most. The reorganization of DNA over the course of the cell's lifetime is linked to its death. But when the cell's DNA is stabilized, both the average lifespan and maximum lifespan increase. A protein that stabilizes the chromosomes of a yeast cell, encoded by a gene of the same name, is called sir2. When an extra copy of Sir2 gene was introduced into a yeast cell, enabling to generate about twice as much sir2 protein and stabilizing the DNA, the yeast lived about 30 percent longer.

Sir2 is believed to be the founding member, in evolutionary terms, of a family of genes known as sirtuins that are present in all complex life forms. The Sir2 gene is activated when the yeast cells are stressed. It in turn acts to stabilize the chromosome, making the cells to live longer. More recently, another gene has been identified that controls Sir2, a master regulator called, PNC1. Stress turns on the PNC1 gene, the activity of which in turn activates Sir2.

There is a set of plant molecules (the sirtuin activating compounds, STACs), which activates the sir2 protein. These molecules act through Sir2, because when that gene is deleted, the effect is vanished. When, STACs are fed to roundworms and flies, they also live longer. It seems that the STACs may be universally efficacious, even in humans.

**The Links between
Sirtuins and CR**

There appears to be a relationship between sirtuins, insulin-signaling pathway and the caloric restriction. The sirtuins are controlled by insulin and another closely related hormone, insulin-like growth factor-1 (IGF-1). In mammals, there is SIRT1 gene (equivalent to Sir2 in yeast) which rises when levels of insulin and IGF-1 fall, as they do in a calorie-restricted organism. When sirtuins are triggered by STACs they do not cause infertility, as occurs with caloric restriction. Thus, with STACs we can get all the benefits of caloric restriction without the trade-offs like infertility.

The Hormesis:
Benefits of Mild Stress

The concept that mild stress might lead to health benefits is called hormesis. Plants given low doses of an herbicide, for example, can actually become stronger and grow better. It is thought that STACs increase lifespan because they are produced by plants when stressed or starving. The plants make these molecules to turn on their own protective sirtuin genes in order to defend themselves.

Resveratrol is a plant extract of 50 percent unknown composition. The molecule is very sensitive to light and air and has a short shelf-life. A high level of resveratrol is present in red wines. The molecule, which is concentrated in the skins of grapes, is insoluble in water. The red wine is made from grapes is processed with their skins, and alcohol is used for extraction. Traditionally, the wine is stored in dark, light-proof bottles, corked to keep oxygen out. Therefore, resveratrol is preserved in red wines.

ROS AND METABOLIC
DYSFUNCTION

ROS and Antioxidants

The free radical theory of ageing is fundamental to the understanding of ageing. We can look at the uncontrolled metabolic dysfunction as a model for accelerated ageing. For example, the obesity is a disturbed metabolic state, having potential to cause metabolic syndrome, in which insulin-resistance leads to diabetes, heart disease and other changes akin to ageing related disorders.

The ROS or free radicals are highly chemically hyper-active molecules. They react with DNA and cellular proteins to oxidise, damage and make them dysfunctional, apart from giving rise to mutations and other abnormalities.

The antioxidants, on the other hand, mop-up free radicals and help in reducing their damaging effects. In the mice experimental studies, the antioxidant effect was obvious in increasing the longevity as well as in preventing morbidity. There was less evidence of heart disease and there occurred fewer cataracts than in normally ageing mice.

Many diseases and infirmities are associated with ageing. By suitably using antioxidants, it is possible to delay or retard the underlying process of ageing. In the studies, taking antioxidant supplements like Vitamin C and E might not have helped, but eating fruits and vegetables rich in antioxidants is known to improve the health.

**The Metabolism and
Oxidative Stress**

The lifespan has been linked to metabolic rate. The metabolism generates free radicals - reactive oxygen species (ROS) - that can damage DNA and proteins. Animals that live fast, die young because a high metabolic rate produces large number of free radicals. According to this theory, long-lived animals should have high concentrations of antioxidant enzymes in their tissues and low concentrations of free radicals.

There is another related theory, which states that metabolic stability is a better predictor of longevity than metabolic rate. It proposes that an organism's ability to maintain stable levels of free radicals is more important than how fast it produces them. According to this the pharmacological agents that simply act to reduce ROS concentrations may even be harmful, because they could perturb the delicate balance necessary for normal cell function.

Accumulation of
Free Radical Damage

The accumulation of free-radical damage may be the key regulator of lifespan. Thus, there may develop ability to resist free-radical damage by genetic alterations in the insulin-signaling pathway. It appears that the gene daf-2 is a potent gene that triggers multiple factors leading to increase the longevity. While some genes downstream from daf-2 encode antioxidant proteins, which protect the body against damage from free radicals, others code for proteins called 'chaperones,' which help in folding the decomposed proteins and taking them to the lysosomal system for digestion, and still other genes encode anti-microbial agents that kill bacteria and fungi, while a set of metabolic genes, when turned down, also promotes longevity.

The improved ability to withstand environmental insults, thus, increases longevity. The metabolic stability is more important than metabolic rate in determining lifespan. In fact, ageing research has shown that long-lived animals are more resistant to pathogens and other environmental stresses.

The correlation between disease-resistance and longevity has led researchers to test the efficacy of sirtuins against various diseases associated with ageing, like Alzheimer's disease and other neuro-degenerative disorders. The sirtuins appear to be pro-survival molecules. Feeding the lab mice resveratrol, a sirtuin-activating compound derived from plants, suppresses the growth of implanted neoplasia and tumours.

Single Nucleotide Polymorphisms
The Impact on Ageing

The results from the New England Centenarian Project point that there is a tendency toward longevity-clusters in population groups. In many centenarians' families, longevity appears to be a dominant trait. Also, that one in 10,000 people alive today has longevity genes.

As human-being, we all have the same genes, but vary from each other based on certain single nucleotide polymorphisms (SNPs). The vast majority of these SNPs have no impact on longevity. But a few of them might increase the likelihood of high cholesterol, cardiovascular disease, or Alzheimer's disease. Negative mutations can accumulate in the course of evolution, as long as they do not affect fertility or lifespan during an organism's reproductive years.

In addition to being free of the negative genetic variations common in other human beings, the centenarians also have some positive mutations that increase the possibility of longer lifespan. In human longevity studies, single nucleotide polymorphism (SNP) analysis identified a large number of genetic variants with metabolic effects[44]. About a hundred of these metabolic manipulations enhance longevity by retarding aging comparable to CR.

Further, the genes work differently in different population groups, depending on environmental influences. A gene that leads to high blood-lipid levels in primitive, physically active, food-limited populations might promote longevity in them, but can cause heart disease and lead to early death in a sedentary modern urban. Nevertheless, the clustering of genetic variations among centenarians suggests that there may be one or two genes common among long-surviving individuals that have a much stronger influence than others.

RELATING LAB RESEARCH TO LONGEVITY IN HUMANS

The prime question is whether the interventions that work in lab animals will work in humans? Extending the lifespan of a fly or a worm or a yeast cell is exciting, but easy because they have just one type of receptor for both insulin and growth hormones. But, in complex animals these pathways diverge: the mammals have separate insulin and insulin-like growth-factor receptors. Although these receptors in mammals are structurally and functionally similar, one is part of a system that regulates metabolism, while the other primarily mediates growth.

The insulin signaling has connections to diabetes and metabolic syndrome. In the experimental mouse, if insulin signaling is knocked out in fat tissue (FIRKO mouse), it remains lean as it ages. The FIRKO mouse is not more active than the wild one. One hypothesis is that the FIRKO mice are metabolically inefficient. The calorie-restricted animals also exhibit an altered metabolism. They are slightly less efficient at converting food into energy, but produce fewer free radicals and so experience less oxidative damage.

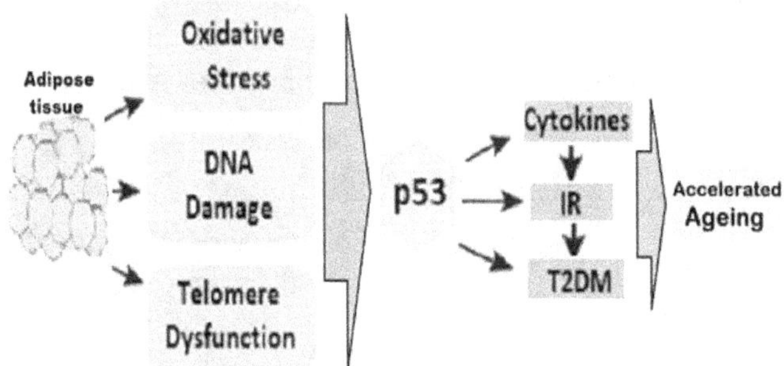

Figure 17: Adiposity, stress factors, metabolic disorders and accelerated ageing

In human muscle, there is a decrease in oxidative metabolism with age. Considering the emerging connections among diabetes, oxidative metabolism, and ageing in muscle and fat, there appears to be a common oxidative pathway that becomes less efficient with age. On the other hand, the links between insulin signaling, caloric restriction, and obesity could be centered on adipose tissue, which secretes hormones called adipokines, may be acting on other tissues to modify ageing (Fig 17). Alternatively, it could be a source of molecules involved in oxidative stress, such as free radicals.

UNDERSTANDING AGEING THROUGH THEORIES OF AGEING

There is a growing interest in phenomenon of ageing. Why and how ageing occurs, is a hot topic in scientific circles. There is search for a general theory to explain of phenomenon of ageing. But the observations derived from various studies are numerous and abundant adding to the confusion. To transform these numerous and diverse observations into a comprehensive body of knowledge, a general theory of ageing and longevity is required. A general theory of ageing may be evolved in the future from synthesis between systems theory (reliability theory) and understanding of derivations based on the evolutionary theories of ageing relying on the biological evolution by natural selection.

The Reliability Theory of Ageing

Ageing can be understood as the summary term for a set of processes, which contribute to pathophysiological deterioration and ultimately to death with the passage of time[45]. These processes contribute to the age-related decline in performance, productivity and health. Here, the failure is an outcome, according to the reliability theory, when the system deviates from optimal anticipated and desired behavior.

The reliability theory holds that a system may deteriorate with age even if it is built from non-aging elements with constant failure rate. The key issue here is the system's redundancy for irreplaceable elements, which is responsible for the ageing phenomenon. There may be no specific underlying elementary ageing process itself - instead ageing may be largely a property of redundant system as a whole.

Reliability Theory in Action

The reliability theory is a general theory of systems failure applied in mechanical engineering setting. This theory can allow us to predict the age-related failure kinetics for a given system and given reliability of its components. Thus:

• Redundancy is a key notion for understanding ageing and the systemic nature of ageing in particular. Systems, which are redundant in numbers of irreplaceable elements, do deteriorate over time (i.e. age), even if they are built of non-ageing elements.

• Paradoxically, the apparent ageing rate or expression of ageing is higher for systems with higher redundancy levels. Redundancy exhaustion over the life course explains the observed mortality convergence at later life as well as the observed late-life mortality deceleration, levelling-off, and mortality plateaus.

• Living organisms seem to be formed with a high load of initial damage, and therefore their lifespan and ageing patterns may be sensitive to early-life conditions that determine this initial damage load during early development.

• Reliability theory explains why mortality rates increase exponentially with age, by taking into account the initial flaws (defects) in newly formed systems.

• Reliability theory helps evolutionary theories to explain how the onset of deleterious outcomes can be postponed by a simple increase in initial redundancy levels. From the reliability perspective, the increase in initial redundancy levels is the simplest way to improve survival particularly at early reproductive ages.

Evolutionary Theories of Ageing

Following are the major evolutionary theories of ageing:

• Mutation accumulation theory,

• Antagonistic pleiotropy theory,

• Disposable soma theory, and

• Theory of programmed death.

At present the most workable evolutionary theories are the mutation accumulation theory and the antagonistic pleiotropy theory. But these theories are not mutually exclusive.

The Basic Tenets of Evolutionary Theories

Evolutionary theories of ageing and longevity try to explain the remarkable differences in observed ageing rates and longevity records across different biological species through interplay between the processes of mutation and selection. There are, though, some puzzling observations in the life cycles of some biological species. For example, a bamboo plant reproduces asexually for about 100 years, forming a dense stand of plants. Then in one season all of the plants flower simultaneously, reproduce sexually, and die. A similar observation is seen in the pacific salmon.

Thus, there has evolved the idea that sexual reproduction may come with a cost for species longevity. Thus, in addition to mutation and selection, the reproductive cost, or, more generally, the trade-offs between different traits of organisms may also contribute to the evolution of species ageing and longevity. The evolutionary theories of ageing are closely related to the genetics of ageing because biological evolution is possible only for heritable manifestations of ageing.

The Darwin's theory is based on the idea of random and heritable variation of biological traits between individuals (caused by mutations) with subsequent natural selection for preferential reproduction of those individuals who are particularly fit to a given environment. It is expected, therefore, that the biological evolution acts to increase the fitness and performance of species evolving in successive generations. From this perspective it is difficult to understand why natural selection leads to senescence and late-life degenerative diseases instead of eternal youth and immortality. In addition, many manifestations of ageing occur after the reproductive period of organisms.

But the ageing and lifespan do evolve in subsequent generations of biological species in a theoretically predicted manner depending on particular living conditions. For example, a selection for later reproduction produced, as expected, longer-lived fruit flies while placing animals in a more dangerous environment with high extrinsic mortality redirected evolution, as predicted, to a shorter lifespan in subsequent generations. The evolutionary theory is, thus, consistent with the plasticity of ageing and longevity.

Evolutionary Theories in Action

The evolutionary theory of ageing may be considered as part of a more general life history theory, which tries to explain how evolution designs organisms to achieve reproductive success and avoid extinction. It answers why some organisms are small or large, why do they mature early or late, why do they have few or many offspring, why do they have a short or a long life, and why must they grow old and die.

Current evolutionary explanations of ageing and limited longevity of biological species are based on following major evolutionary theories:

• <u>Mutation accumulation theory</u>: From the evolutionary perspective, ageing is an inevitable result of the declining force of natural selection with age. Over successive generations, late-acting deleterious mutations will accumulate, leading to an increase in mortality rates late in life. This particular evolutionary theory, considers ageing a by-product of natural selection.

According to this theory, persons loaded with a deleterious mutation have fewer chances to reproduce if the deleterious effect of this mutation is expressed earlier in life. By contrast, people expressing a mutation at older ages can reproduce before the illness occurs, such as the case with familial Alzheimer's disease. This prediction was tested through the analysis of genealogical data on familial longevity in European royal and noble families, data well known for their reliability and accuracy. It was found that the regression slope for the dependence of offspring lifespan on parental lifespan increases with parental lifespan, exactly as predicted by the mutation accumulation theory.

• <u>Antagonistic pleiotropy theory</u>: Late-acting deleterious genes may even be favoured by selection and be actively accumulated in populations if they have any beneficial effects early in life. This is currently the most accepted theory of ageing[46].

An example of antagonistic pleiotropy refers to replicative cellular senescence (cell division limit), which is known to suppress tumorigenesis by switching cells into a state of arrested growth. This very process that suppresses tumorigenesis early in life, however, may promote cancer in later life because senescent cells stimulate other premalignant and malignant cells to proliferate and to form tumours. Here again there is a trade-off between the earlier protective effect of growth arrest because of cellular senescence and the later detrimental effect caused by cancer promotion.

The antagonistic pleiotropy theory also explains why reproduction may come with a cost for species longevity and may even induce death, as in bamboo plants and pacific salmon. Indeed, any mutations favouring more intensive reproduction (more offspring produced) will be propagated in future generations even if these mutations have some deleterious effects in later life. For example, mutations causing overproduction of sex hormones may increase the sex drive, libido, reproductive efforts, and success, and therefore they may be favoured by selection despite causing prostate cancer (in males) and ovarian cancer (in females) later in life. Thus, the idea of reproductive cost, or more generally of trade-offs, between different traits of the organism follows directly from antagonistic pleiotropy theory.

These predictions were tested. By postponing reproduction to later ages, the intensity of selection on the later stages of life was increased. This selection for late reproduction increased lifespan of the selected populations. Interestingly, the increase in longevity was accompanied by an evolutionary decline in fertility early in adult life, confirming the prediction of the antagonistic pleiotropy theory.

These two theories of ageing, namely mutation accumulation theory and antagonistic pleiotropy theory are not mutually exclusive. In fact, both evolutionary mechanisms may operate at the same time. The main difference between the two theories is that in the mutation accumulation theory, genes with negative effects at old age accumulate passively from one generation to the next while in the antagonistic pleiotropy theory, these genes are actively kept in the gene pool by selection.

• <u>Disposable soma theory</u>: Most researchers agree that the disposable soma theory is a modified and narrowly defined variant of the antagonistic pleiotropy theory of ageing. A key assumption in the disposable soma theory of ageing is that mothers trade off their own somatic maintenance against investment in offspring[47]. This trade-off by mothers affects the ageing in offspring in terms of accumulated damage, as indicated by oxidative stress or telomere length.

• <u>Weismann's Theory of Programmed Death</u>: Weismann proposed in 1882 that aging was an evolved genetically programmed adaptation that had a species benefit. It states that there exists a specific death mechanism designed by natural selection to eliminate the old, and therefore worn-out, members of a population. The purpose of this programmed death of the old is to clean up the living space and to free up resources for younger generations. Further, as per this theory, the ageing appears to be one of a number of related and interactive life-cycle characteristics including age-at-puberty suggesting that it might be controlled by such biological mechanisms[48]. Presently, this theory is not taken seriously.

Suggesting the theory of programmed death, Weismann came to an idea that there is a specific limitation on the number of times a somatic cell can divide. Years late, the concept of cell division limit, became known as the Hayflick limit.

IMPLICATIONS OF THEORIES OF AGEING

Numerous studies demonstrate that several manifestations of ageing can be postponed or even reversed, and that lifespan can be significantly extended in experimental animals. The studies have outlined remarkable plasticity of ageing and longevity and a significant potential for further extension of human lifespan.

On this basis we begin to think of ageing as a disorder that can be cured, or at least postponed. Research in the field of ageing holds unlimited promises of slowing ageing and increasing longevity along with better health.

The theories of ageing are important because they open new opportunities for research by suggesting testable predictions. In fact, the field of ageing research has been completely transformed in the past decades.

CHAPTER ELEVEN

TAMING PROAGEING PATHWAYS:
Modifying Metabolic Disequilibrium and Oxidative Stress

IDENTIFYING PRO-AGEING PATHWAYS

The Ageing and Lifespan

The unicellular and multicellular organisms, both, age chronologically with their life span representing the average age of the organisms at death. At cellular level, the chronological ageing is mediated in part by ROS generated by mitochondria and attended by loss of mitochondrial function. In case of unicellular organisms like yeast (Saccharomyces), the number of times a yeast mother cell divides to produce daughter cells in its lifetime represents the replicative life span. With the cell survival and growth, there occurs progressive accumulation of ribosomal DNA circles in the nucleolus, which has been related to the replicative ageing.

Ageing is a major risk factor for disease-states such as atherosclerosis and cardiovascular disease, degenerative disorders including neurodegenerative diseases and disorders due to altered cellular physiology and division like cancer. Understanding the ageing phenomenon leads to biological insights that identify potential interventions to slow down the ageing process. The ageing, thus, becomes a modifiable risk factor and leads to the expectant possibility to extend the lifespan. Through targeted lifestyle changes and potentially effective interventions through nutraceuticals and pharmaceuticals it may be possible to reduce the age-related chronic and debilitating morbidities and improve the health-span.

Ageing Mechanisms and Pathways

Apparently, there are similarities between the pathways that regulate stress resistance, cellular protection, and ageing in lower animals like C. elegans, yeast and Drosophila as well as in mammals. Insulin and insulin-like signaling factors regulate survival and lifespan and play a significant role in longevity in various animal species, from nematodes and Drosophila to higher vertebrates. Apart from this, the Akt and Ras pathways playing an important role in IGF-1 (insulin-like growth factor 1) signaling, appear to regulate ageing in mammals. In fact, Ras, Akt and Serine/threonine-protein kinase (Sgk-1) play an essential role in cellular functions and metabolism and may accelerate ageing in some tissues and organs.

The discovery of the role of Ras (Ras proteins), adenylate cyclase, PKA (protein kinase A), and Sod (Superoxide dismutase) in the regulation of stress resistance and longevity, and the role of the IGF-1-like pathway in ageing both in Saccharomyces and C. elegans have outlined the mechanisms and pathways that control chronological ageing in simpler organisms like Saccharomyces and C. elegans. These regulatory pathways and mechanisms share similarities and include members of the PKB (Protein kinase B, also known as Akt), family of serine-threonine kinases and stress resistance transcription factors controlling the antioxidant enzymes and heat shock proteins. Similar pathways and mechanisms including the IGF-1-like receptor, Akt and a stress resistance transcription factor are also responsible for longevity regulation in Drosophila. Further, certain mutations, periods of starvation and dietary calorie restriction activate these pathways in Saccharomyces, C. elegans and Drosophila.

Further up along the evolution, the role of IGF-1 and Insulin signaling in the regulation of the mouse life span, together with the central role of the Akt and Ras pathways in IGF-1 signaling, indicates that mechanisms may regulate stress resistance and ageing in mammals. In fact, Ras, Akt and Sgk-1 may accelerate ageing in various cells but at the same time play an essential role in functions like cell metabolism, growth, and division. Various studies document that the mice lacking serum IGF-1, Drosophila deficient in IGF-1-like signaling, and Saccharomyces lacking the Akt/PKB homolog Sch9 live longer but are smaller in size. On the other hand, Saccharomyces lacking RAS2 (a gene encoding Ras) and C. elegans with mutations involving daf-2 (the gene encoding the insulin-like/IGF-1 tyrosine kinase receptor) are able to attain normal size and live longer.

Insulin/IGF-1 and Allied Pathways

The studies in C. elegans, Drosophila and mice point to the insulin/IGF-1/phosphatidylinositol-3-kinase (PI3K)/Akt-like pathway being the prime regulators of ageing and longevity. The insulin/IGF-1 pathway, which is a complex signal transduction pathway, includes an IGF-1-like receptor, PI3K, members of the Akt/protein kinase B (PKB) kinases and Forkhead transcription factor. The studies indicate that the components of an IGF-1-like pro-ageing pathway are conserved from Saccharomyces to mammals. Further, in C. elegans serum- and glucocorticoid-inducible kinase (SGK-1), playing an important role in longevity regulation, has a 55% sequence analogy to Akt3. In Saccharomyces, a similar pathway, which includes Sch9, a serine-threonine kinase homologous to mammalian Akt/protein kinase B, appears to regulate lifespan and longevity.

Further, in Saccharomyces, C. elegans and Drosophila, the partially conserved glucose or insulin/IGF-1-like pathways down-regulate antioxidant activity, reduce the accumulation of glycogen or fat, and improve growth and decrease longevity. It has been shown that the mutations impairing activity of these pathways extend longevity. In mammals, IGF-1 appears to activate the signal transduction pathways analogous to the longevity regulatory pathways in C. elegans and Drosophila and decrease longevity (Fig 18).

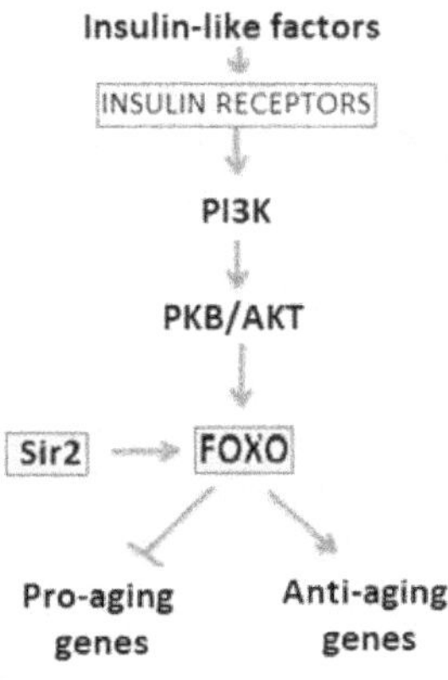

Figure 18. Insulin-like peptides activate insulin receptors, which phosphorylate the enzyme PI3K. The phosphorylate PI3K recruits protein kinase B. PKB signals inhibit FOXO to negatively regulate expression of pro-aging genes and to positively express anti-aging genes. The Sir2 increases longevity by influencing FOXO.

In humans, alterations resulting in deficiency of plasma GH or IGF-1 cause dwarfism and obesity and may negatively the chronological lifespan.

The Ras Dependent Pathways

The chronological ageing in Saccharomyces, in addition, is also regulated by a second pathway that includes Ras, adenylate cyclase, protein kinase A, the transcription factors - Msn2 and Msn4 (multicopy suppressor of SNF1 mutation proteins 2 and 4), and Sod2. This pathway is partially influenced by Sch9, has been shown to have impact on stress resistance and life span in Saccharomyces. Ras and Sch9 function in overlapping manner to stimulate growth but impair stress resistance.

The Ras is highly conserved in various organisms from Saccharomyces to humans and it appears that Ras proteins through mammalian IGF-1 signaling, accelerate ageing in mammals. Further, the pro-ageing effect of the Ras/cAMP/PKA pathway through activation of PKA leads to decreased lifespan. On the other hand, the Ras inactivation via increasing Sod activity, leads to survival benefit and increased lifespan in Saccharomyces, C. elegans and Drosophila, as well as mammalian neuronal cells, in vitro.

THE PROAGING Vs.
LONGEVITY MECHANISMS

Ras Pathway and its Interrelationship

There are similarities in the pathways regulating oxidative stress and longevity in Saccharomyces, C. elegans and Drosophila. It appears that similar mechanisms influence cell survival and aging in mammals. The four Saccharomyces genes, SOD1, SOD2, RAS2 and SCH9 have been found to have profound effect on its chronological lifespan and are conserved from Saccharomyces to Homo Sapiens.

The Ras exhibits contradictory pro- and anti-ageing effects on cellular physiology. Thus, depending on ROS and other factors, Ras may either prevent apoptosis to promote cell growth and function or induce cellular damage and senescence. The chronic Ras-dependent increase in the generation of oxidants appears to increase cellular appendicular damage, accelerate ageing, and contribute to age-related disorders[49].

IGF and Insulin Like Factors

Insulin and insulin-like signaling (IIS) regulate survival and lifespan and play a significant role in longevity in a variety of animal species, from C. elegans and Drosophila to higher vertebrates and mammals[50]. Several genes of the somatotropic axis act as longevity determinants, and the variants of FOXO3A, downstream signaling molecule in the insulin/IGF pathway, are associated with extreme longevity in humans. Finally, several functional mutations of the human IGF-IR have been discovered in centenarians.

The insulin signaling is primarily involved in nutrient regulation, whereas IGF-1 modulates growth. Various studies have linked the IIS pathway to the ageing process. Further, the genetic alterations modestly reducing IIS signaling positively influence the lifespan[51]. In mice experiments, reduced circulating IGF-1 levels contributed to a 16% increase in median lifespan of female GH mutant mice, but a similar deletion in male mice did not alter lifespan. The underlying physiology of this sexual dimorphic response, however, is not well understood.

Sirtuins and Other Key Proteins

Several key proteins in the evolutionary conserved pathways belonging to the sirtuin family of NAD-dependent enzymes, apart from components of the insulin/IGF2 pathway, mechanistic target and downstream effectors of mTOR kinase, have been linked to regulation of lifespan. There are seven sirtuins, SIRT1 to 7, existing in various cellular compartments in mammals. The SIRT1, SIRT6, and SIRT7 are predominantly nuclear forms, whereas SIRT3, SIRT4 and SIRT5 are present in mitochondria.

The sirtuins catalyse various deacylation reactions including demalonylation, desuccinylation and deproprionylation at cellular level. The link of these enzymes to ageing was noted when it was observed that overexpression of Sir2 extended replicative lifespan in S. cerevisiae. In an important development, the life-extending benefit of caloric restriction in Saccharomyces has been linked to Sir2. Further, similar to higher organisms, the overexpression of Sir2 in both C. elegans and Drosophila is able to extend lifespan. The lifespan extending effects of sirtuins has been linked to favourable alterations in genomic stability, mitochondrial function and biogenesis, and suppression of inflammation[52].

A polyphenol, resveratrol is the sirtuin-activating molecule which has been documented to improve the lifespan in Saccharomyces, C. elegans and Drosophila. In mice models and clinical studies in humans, resveratrol appears to protect from metabolic disorders and various age-related diseases associated with physiological ageing and diet-induced obesity[53]. The manipulation of sirtuin activity through sirtuin-activating compounds (STACs) is, thus, holds promise to improve various aspects of cellular physiology (Fig 19).

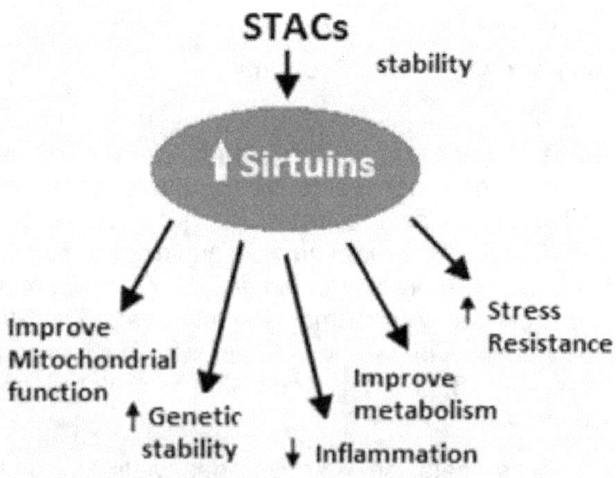

Figure 19: Protective role of STACs in cellular physiology

mTOR (mechanistic Target of Rapamycin) Signaling

The mTOR kinase is a serine/threonine protein kinase belonging to the PI3K-related family, inhibited by rapamycin, an immunosuppressive drug. Working as an energy sensor in the simple organisms like C. elegans, it is activated by surplus nutrients supply. On activation, mTOR inhibits catabolic processes like autophagy and promotes anabolic processes like protein synthesis and ribosomal biogenesis to promote cellular growth and proliferation. The limited availability of nutrients or forced caloric restriction inhibits mTOR and promotes autophagy and halts proliferation. The mTOR inhibition has been linked to the ability of the cell or tissue to withstand energetic, oxidative and hypoxic stresses, improve mitochondrial biogenesis and physiology, activation of autophagy and improvement of stem cell self-renewal[54].

In mammals, mTOR exists as mTOR complex 1 (mTORC1) and mTOR complex 2 (mTORC2).. While mTORC1 regulates cell growth and metabolism, mTORC2 instead controls proliferation and survival primarily by phosphorylating several members of the AGC (PKA/PKG/PKC) family of protein kinases[55].

THE INTERACTIONS BETWEEN LONGEVITY PATHWAYS

In general, the three pathways - sirtuins, mTOR and the IIS responding to nutrient availability, modulate the lifespan. The major interconnection between these pathways is through AMP-activated protein kinase (AMPK). The mTOR activity declines and sirtuin activity increases on exposure to starvation or caloric restriction. The activated AMPK influences intracellular metabolism and upregulates NAD+ levels and SIRT1 activity. The SIRT1 in turn deacetylate and regulate FOXO activity. The interaction between AMPK and the sirtuins is bidirectional.

The three longevity pathways, sirtuins, IIS and mTOR, also converge to regulate autophagy through multiple interdependent effectors. The ISS inhibits autophagy through activating PI3K/AKT signaling. ThePI3K/AKT in turn stimulates mTOR. The AKT activation has a negatively impact on FOXO transcriptional activity, whereas FOXO regulates the expression of various autophagic genes. The sirtuins influence the FOXO activity through deacetylation and modulate autophagic flux, similar to IIS and mTOR32. In addition, SIRT1 also deacetylate autophagy genes and regulate autophagic flux. The SIRT1/FOXO pathway is critical for the CR-induced autophagy response.

In addition, there is a synergy for the positive feedback loop involving AMPK and FOXO proteins, suggesting that the complex interactions between these pathways are dynamic.

METABOLIC DISEQUILIBRIUM, DISEASE AND AGEING

Metabolic Disorders and Ageing Process

There is increasing evidence that metabolic disequilibrium and disorders influence the ageing process, prevalence of various diseases and survival including the QOL. The role of master-switch and genomic guardian, p53 is important in this context. With weight gain and obesity, the adipose tissue mediates various metabolic disorders such as insulin resistance (IR), metabolic syndrome (MetS), dyslipidemia and type 2 diabetes mellitus (T2DM), which accelerate the ageing process in various tissues and organs through a number of metabolic pathways and negatively affect the lifespan.

The development of IR is one of the most important risk factors for metabolic diseases in the middle aged and elderly. The decline in lean body mass and increase in body fat, particularly visceral adiposity, often accompany ageing and contribute to the development of IR. The ageing process correlates with β-cell functional decline, decreased β-cell proliferation capacity and enhanced sensitivity to apoptosis. With ageing, there occurs altered mitochondrial function in various tissues, including skeletal muscle, which can lead to oxidative damage of macromolecules, including nuclear and mitochondrial DNA (mtDNA). The mitochondrial oxidative and phosphorylation functions are reduced by about 40 percent, along with increased intramyocellular and intrahepatocellular lipid content and decreased insulin-stimulated glucose uptake. The mitochondrial theory of ageing posits that mitochondrial dysfunction may be a fundamental cause of cellular senescence and apoptosis.

Metabolic Syndrome and Visceral Adiposity

The MetS is directly related to the accumulation of visceral adiposity in middle age associated with overnutrition and sedentary lifestyle. In addition, there may be a genetic predisposition to MetS. Apart from, insulin, two other hormones associated with development of MetS, are leptin and adiponectin which are produced by adipose tissue. The leptin levels are proportional to amount of adiposity and have anorectic effect and enhance metabolism. With adiposity, there occurs resistance to leptin effects due to hypertriglyceridemia. Adiponectin enhances insulin sensitivity and decreases triglycerides levels, but a low level of adiponectin accompanies the development of IR. The visceral fat (VF) is associated with increased cytokines such as interleukin-6 (IL-6) and tumor-necrosis factor α (TNF-α), which play a major role in development of IR[56]. With obesity, the p53 is activated in adipose tissue leading to inflammation and insulin resistance culminating into T2DM (Fig 20).

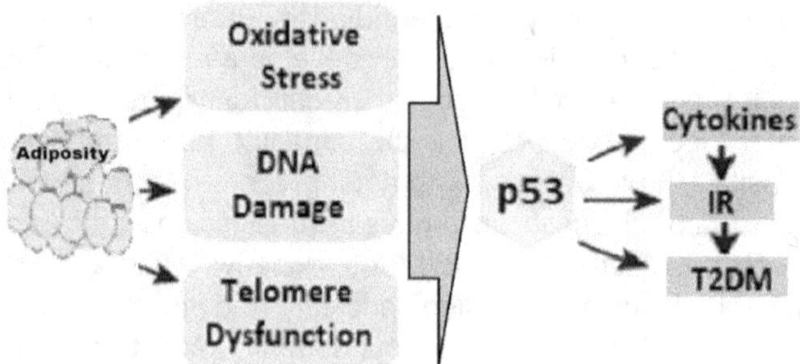

Figure 20: Adiposity, Stress Factors, p53 and genesis of Metabolic Disorders

In animal models, the inhibition of p53 activity in adipose tissue ameliorated the senescence-like changes, decreased the expression of pro-inflammatory cytokines and improved insulin resistance in mice with T2DM-like disease[57].

The Regulator Role of p53

The p53 is a 53-k dalton molecule, hence the name. It has been called the guardian of genome. It regulates the cell cycle, functions as tumor suppressor and plays an important role in apoptosis, genomic stability, and inhibition of angiogenesis. In normal cell p53 is in inactive form by its binding with mdm2. The various stressors lead to dissociation of the p53 and mdm2 complex. The p53 activation in adipose tissue is a pro-ageing signal, with negative influence on longevity (Fig 21).

Metabolic Link to Ageing, Obesity and Diabetes

Ageing, as such, is characterized by deterioration in the maintenance of homeostatic processes over time, leading to functional decline and increased risk for disease. Metabolically, the ageing process is associated with IR, changes in body composition and physiological decline in growth hormone (GH), insulin-like growth factor-1 (IGF -

1), and sex steroids. There occurs mitochondrial decline and endoplasmic membrane abnormalities with ageing.

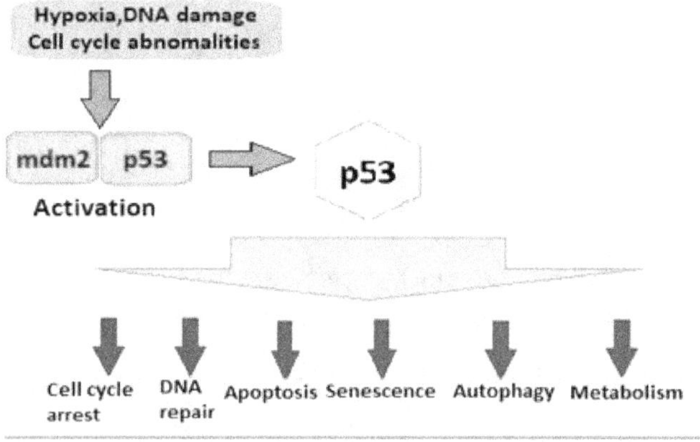

Fig 21: The stress factors activate p53 by dissociating the mdm2-p53 complex, which influences cell cycle, metabolism, DNA repair, senescence, apoptosis and autophagy and aging process.

Further, there is an ageing, obesity, and diabetes link. The physiological and histological changes in ageing organs have been associated with oxidative stress, disruption of homeo-static pathways, genetic instability and telomere shortening. Diabetes, too, accelerates ageing through certain complex mechanisms, which include inflammatory pathways. With age, there is a decrease in subcutaneous fat (SF) and increase in VF, which is associated with metabolic dysfunction, IR and development of T2DM. Adipose tissue from diabetic shows senescence-like changes.

The studies have linked MetS and obesity to tendency for cognitive functional decline. These patients are more likely to have small infarcts and develop vascular dementia as occurs in hypertensive patients. The IR-associated hyperglycemia per se produces cognitive dysfunction. The MetS and T2DM, both, predispose to Alzheimer's disease.

Skeletal muscle loss or sarcopenia is a major contributor to frailty with ageing. On the other hand, the proinflammatory state associated with ageing and obesity leads to sarcopenia. It represents an unfavourable phenotypic change associated with ageing and linked to a reduction in energy expenditure and exacerbation of IR[58]. The IR leads to further decline in muscle quantity and quality, reduced skeletal muscle strength, and accelerated skeletal muscle loss.

Adiposity, Altered Metabolism and Ageing

There is increasing evidence that mammalian ageing is influenced, in part, by adiposity[59]. The ageing, visceral fat and inflammation increase risk of metabolic diseases like obesity, IR, T2DM, CVD and HTN. The WAT mediates various age-associated metabolic disorders such as IR and dyslipidemia which can negatively affect the lifespan. The sirtuins and CR through Sirt1 appears to regulate WAT by repressing p53.

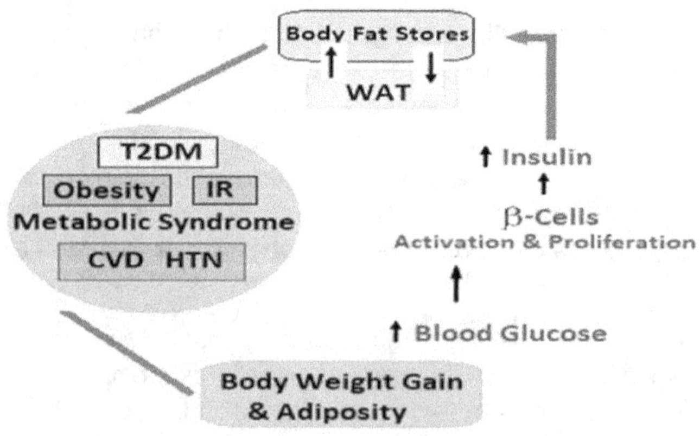

Figure 22: Metabolic Changes triggered by adiposity.

The WAT, muscle, liver, and pancreatic β cells are integrated in a regulatory circuit (Fig 22). Chronic high food intake triggers an increase in blood glucose. The surges in blood glucose will activate β cells to produce more insulin, in the long run leading to β cell proliferation and ultimately failure. Insulin signals WAT to store fat as triglycerides. The triglycerides store influences the levels of hormones produced by the WAT cells, primarily increase in leptin and a decrease in adiponectin, which influence the insulin sensitivity of metabolic organs.

THE CALORIC RESTRCTION: CONCEPTS, BASIS AND PRACTICE

Nutritional Needs in Older Adults

The energy needs of individuals are determined by their body composition, especially the fat free lean mass and level of physical activity. Most older adults lose fat free mass as they age, with skeletal muscle being lost at a rate of approximately 1% per year in the over 70s[60]. They are increasingly less physically active and has a sedentary nature of activity of daily living (ADL). Therefore, older adults have lower requirements for energy. Further, there is a change in nutritional needs during the middle age and later when no actual growth is taking place, though there is an increased need of nutrients to take care of increased wear and tear with age.

The diet-gene interaction is a major determinant of health and illness. The extra calorie intake causes nutritional overload and giving rise to adiposity culminating as weight gain and obesity, leading to IR, MetS, T2DM and other metabolic alterations. At the subcellular and cellular level there is increased propensity to damaging effects of reactive oxygen species (ROS).

The calorie restriction or caloric restriction (CR) is a dietary intervention to reduce food intake without incurring malnutrition or nutrient deficiency. The CR has been generally defined as consumption of nutritious diet that is about 40% less in calories compared to ad libitum diet. An optimal food intake and caloric restriction with adequate nutrition (CRAN), in general, promotes health, metabolic homeostasis, disease protection and longevity. The focus of positive lifestyle changes is often on a intake of healthy diet and enhance physical activity; resorting to CR or CRAN is going a step further.

Physiological Effects of Calorie Restricted Diet

Several metabolic and genetic pathways have been identified that govern food ingestion, metabolism, and life span. Various studies in yeast, fruit fly, nematodes like C elegans, rodent models and primates (including Homo sapiens) endorse that a diet adequately fulfilling nutritional needs, but low in calories may improve health and extend the life span[61]. At the physiological level, the effects of CR are very well characterized, beginning with an acute phase upon imposition of the diet followed by an adaptive period of several weeks to reach a stable, altered physiological state, characterised by lower body temperature, lower blood glucose and insulin levels, and reduced body fat and weight. The CR animals also appear to be more resistant to external stressors, including heat and oxidative stress.

One of the most striking features of CR is that it appears to forestall or prevent various late-onset disorders and diseases. For example, CR extends life span in certain lab strains of mice which normally would die of cancer. Thus, CR extends the shortened life span of p53−/− mice which otherwise die of early cancers[62]. CR also extends life span in Fischer rats, which normally die of kidney disease.

Further, CR has been shown efficacious in mouse models of a variety of diseases.

The CR Mechanisms and Pathways

The benefits of CR are not a passive result of lower caloric intake but the consequence of an active regulatory intervention mimicking the food scarcity activating certain genetic and metabolic programs that result in beneficial vital effects. Various genetic and molecular studies in model organisms suggest that CR is a regulated process, in which the SIRT gene plays an important role. The findings suggest that the SIR2 ortholog, Sirt1 in mammals may mediate a broad array of physiological effects that occur in animals on a CR diet. The SIRT1 figures prominently in the redistribution of resources during CR from growth, metabolism and reproduction to maintenance and survival. In the mammals there are at least seven sirtuins (SIRT1-7), each sirtuin influences diverse aspects of the metabolism and biological function.

The CR appears to have physiological benefits through the following mechanisms:

1. CR lowers the core body temperature: An adaptive response to reduce energy expenditure when nutrients availability is curtailed. Lowering the temperature may prolong the lifespan of cold-blooded animals. Mice, which are warm blooded, have been genetically modified to have a reduced core body temperature which increases the lifespan independently of CR.

2. Hormesis: The CR is a low-intensity biological stressor. The CR diet imposes a low-intensity biological stress on the organism to elicit a defensive response that help to protect from disorders of ageing. The CR places the organism in a defensive state to survive in adverse life

situations, resulting in improved health and longer life through activation of longevity genes.

3. Hormonal alterations: Prolonged severe CR lowers total serum and free testosterone while increasing sex hormone binding globulin concentrations in humans. CR increases DHEA in primates, but not in post-pubescent primates. These effects are independent of adiposity. By lowering of the concentration of insulin and insulin-like growth factor 1 and growth hormone, CR has been shown to up-regulate autophagy, the repair mechanism of the cell.

4. CR reduces production of ROS and damage by ROS and promotes adaptations to protect against exogenous radicals. The sublethal mitochondrial stress with ROS initiates beneficial alterations in cellular physiology. In mice, CR slows aging, decreases ROS production and reduces the accumulation of oxidative DNA damage in multiple organs.

5. CR has impact on Sirtuins. Sir2 has been implicated in the ageing of S. cerevisiae and is evolutionary conserved. A study in yeast found that deletions of Sir2 decreased lifespan and its additional copies increased lifespan[63]. In fact, the Sir2 homologs have been identified in a wide range of organisms from bacteria to humans.

6. The results akin to CR, can be achieved with pharmacologic approach by using CR Mimetics, such as rapamycin, via mTOR signaling blockade, resveratrol, by activating SIRT1 activity, and metformin, which stimulates of AMPK activity. Activating SIRT1 pathway appears to be beneficial in preventing some manifestations of ageing (Fig 23).

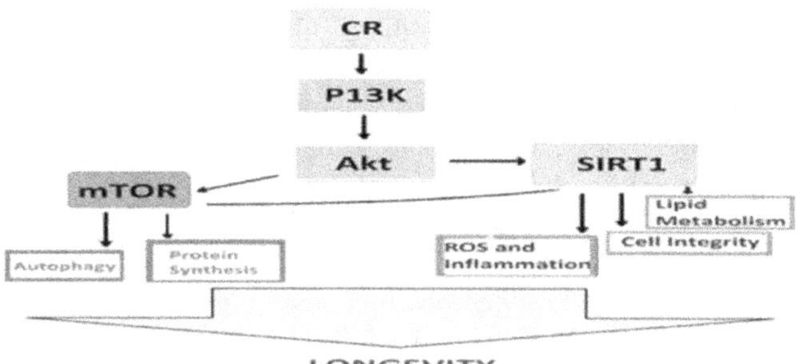

Figure 23. CR, SIRT1 and Life Span: Projected Metabolic Pathways

The CR triggers a more efficient use of glucose via an increase in respiration, analogous to a known metabolic shift that occurs in mammals during CR, in whom there is a transition in muscle cells from using glucose towards the use of fatty acids. This metabolic shift spares glucose for the brain and correlates with the characteristic enhancement of insulin sensitivity in muscle and liver. The resveratrol and CR did not synergize to further extend the life span, suggesting that CR and resveratrol act through the same pathway[64].

The Metabolic Alterations with CR

1. <u>Upregulation of Mitochondrial Uncoupling Proteins</u>: There is a positive correlation between oxygen consumption, i.e., metabolic rate, and life span. The mice on CR have more uncoupled mitochondria than controls, apparently due to upregulation of mitochondrial uncoupling proteins by CR[65]. Because of decreased proton leakage, this would avoid hyperpolarization of the mitochondrial membrane and generate a lower level of ROS.

2. <u>CR and Stress Resistance</u>: CR is known to increase the resistance to oxidative stress, which leads to a greater ability to detoxify ROS and repair oxidative damage, and

slow down cellular decay. Further, the connection between Sirt1 and stress resistance is extensive and Sirt1 appears to target various cellular processes, resulting in a higher threshold for apoptosis.

3. <u>CR and Lipid metabolism</u>: CR modifies favourably the metabolic Changes Triggered by Adiposity. It causes the lipolysis of triglycerides in WAT and the release of free fatty acids, which are taken up and oxidized by metabolic organs. Further, CR increases levels of Sirt1, which modulates the genes concerned with fat storage and hormones. The changes in Sirt1 during long-term CR, by increasing β oxidation of fatty acids and lowering free fatty acids, improve insulin sensitivity and decrease IR (Fig 24).

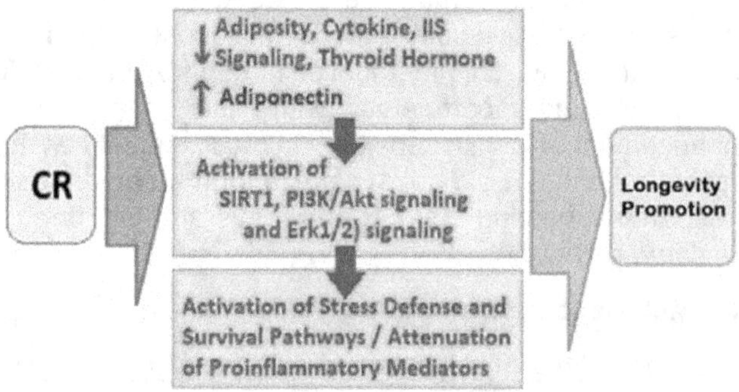

Figure 24. CR and alteration of cellular pathways and circuits

4. <u>CR and Neurodegeneration</u>: In certain mouse models of neurodegenerative diseases, such as Parkinson's or Alzheimer's, CR has been reported to reduce age-associated neuronal loss. CR has also been reported to slow declines in psychomotor and special memory tasks, preserve dendritic spines involved in learning, and improve the plasticity and ability of self-repair of the brain[66].

The Impact of CR on Health and Disease

The state of nutrition influences the aging process and thus, the life span and life expectancy. In addition, CR with adequate nutrition (CRAN) exerts beneficial effects due to numerous metabolic alterations in retarding various disease processes. Both CR and CRMs trigger an adaptive response similar to mild-stress or a low-dose response, referred to as hormesis and influence the biochemical pathways involved in an organism's survival and longevity.

Further, the effects of CR on ageing process and lifespan are applicable to virtually all species. An optimal CR and CRAN reduce the incidence of virtually all diseases of ageing such as cancer, CVD, diabetes, osteoporosis, auto-immune disorders, cognitive decline and neurodegenerative disorders like senile dementia and Alzheimer's disease.

CHAPTER TWLEVE

THE POCKETS OF LONGEVITY:
World of Centenarians and Super-centenarians

The inherent pessimism in human nature, which takes the old age for granted, may try to dismiss the concept and possibility of slowing the ageing and achieving a significant longevity. But the ageless search for the secrets to longevity has inspired recent studies that overturn myths and offer promising visions. The pockets of longevity around the world, too, are an eloquent reminder that the dream can be realized. Further, the longevity trends exist without much scientific intervention. We can very well imagine the impact of advances in science and technology here.

THE REAL VISIONS

FROM 'LOST HORIZON'

The southwestern Chinese people of Pinghan and surrounding Bama County, nestled deep in a remote region surrounded by limestone hills, have the highest percentage of centenarians and super-centenarians in the world. The people of Okinawa, the southern-most region in the Japanese archipelago, also live long lives. The average life expectancy is 81.8 years, many of them live over 100.

The Hunza Valley, sheltered in the northern mountains of Pakistan, is a place of pristine beauty and fosters longevity. Another Asian region is a rural cluster in Sunchang county located in South Korea's mountainous southwest, where many of the local farmers defy ageing and continue to do work in the fields well into their 90s. Elsewhere in Asia there are other, similar pockets of longevity, where for reasons not fully understood, life expectancy exceeds global norms by wide margins.

SECRETS OF ASIAN POCKETS OF LONGEVITY

There are no magic potions, wonder drugs or intricate regimens that bestow longevity. It is invariably the total package that counts: diet, exercise, mental attitude, family and societal support, and the genetic makeup.

Lifestyle Factors

• Diet

The secrets are simple and straight. Eating less is inculcated in their habit through the culture. The Okinawan phrase '*hara* hachi bu', meaning eating less than what makes you full, is a simple but golden saying. The scientific studies have already been steadily advocating this in form of caloric restriction for years giving credence to this simple adage. A daily diet restricted to between half and three-quarters of average recommended 2100 calories, appears to boost health and longevity in humans.

The Okinawans get most of their protein from fish, which provides another so-called good fat: omega-3. This oil is particularly prevalent in fish such as salmon, tuna and mackerel, whose heart-protecting properties are established. Okinawans have about 20 percent incidence of heart attacks as compared to North Americans. Further, when they suffer, they are twice as likely to survive.

The dietary moderation is a consistent feature in their diet. Protein and animal fat typically play a low role. In fact, low fat content is a key factor towards longevity. The eating habits influenced by scarcity appear to contribute to health and longevity. The residents of Bama are not starving, but for most time in the year, they are not full either. In Okinawa, the subjects eat about 20 percent fewer calories than the Japanese average, which is about 20 percent lower than the U.S. average. A calorie-restricted diet might reduce the harmful effects of free radicals - molecules that are generated naturally in the body during biochemical reactions and can damage cells. The free radicals have been implicated with many deleterious effects associated with ageing, including cancers and cardio-vascular diseases.

The researchers are trying to pinpoint particular types of foods consumed in these regions. The people of Bama, for example, cook with oils derived from hemp and tea bush fruits. These oils are rich in unsaturated fat, vitamin E and vitamin B1, the antioxidant nutrients believed to contribute to a healthy cardiovascular system as well as helping prevent certain types of cancers. Similarly, the Okinawans do most of their stir-frying with canola oil, which has been widely shown to protect the body against free radicals.

The prevalence of cancer is similarly low. In Okinawa, breast cancer is five times lower and prostate cancer is seven times lower than in the U.S. This is attributed to in part to Okinawans' very high intake of substances called flavonoids, the   plant-derived compounds that appear to help prevent cancer by neutralizing the destructive effect of free radicals. Okinawa's national dish is a stir-fry called *chample*, which is made from tofu, *goya* - a variety of bitter gourd, and soya beans, which are rich in flavonoids as well as other compounds like isoflavones, saponins and vitamins B and C that provide protection against free radicals. Eating vegetables and fruits is important part of their diet.

But the inhabitants of Okinawa and Hunza Valley, especially the younger generation, are now falling to fantasy of western and fast food. They are succumbing to potato chips, white sugar, and other things. The consequence is the rise in incidence of hypertension, heart attacks and cancer, just like elsewhere.

• Physical Activity

The older people from the Asian oasis of longevity keep physically active. Often engage in hard work in fields and elsewhere to earn their livelihood.

A moderate use of alcohol, no or less smoking, and positive-coping mechanisms are important determinants of longevity.

• The Positive Mind-set

An important prerequisite for longevity is the mind-set - the emotional setup that enables one to cope with stresses of daily living. Inner strength derives in part from vigorous activities, mental as well as physical. The social status and respect are important in building the inner strength, which is the key for achieving a long life.

• Social and Emotional Support

The stable marriage helps in achieving longevity. The social status of elders in Asian societies has been identified as a defining factor in determining a person's longevity.

• The genetic makeup

The longer living Asians appear to have something special in their constitution. They rarely fall ill or suffer from a major disease. It appears that they carry a single gene or a group-of-genes, which have protective effect.

Further, the genetic factor is most important in longevity is proved by the fact that women live longer than men[67]. In general, they have a lifespan five and seven years longer than men. In Okinawa, as many as 86 percent of the centenarians, are female. The women have a genetic advantage. The men can improve their chances for a long life by avoiding destructive social behaviours and habits like smoking and heavy drinking.

<u>The Study of Longevity</u>

Trends in Ashkenazi Jews

A study of over 200 centenarians Ashkenazi Jews and their families, has found that most of them had a mother or a grandfather who lived over 100. There was something that was protecting them despite the fact that many of them did not exercise and were non-vegetarians; some smoked heavily and some had overweight and obesity.

In many of them, the researchers have identified a gene that boosts the size of the lipoproteins. Thus, the protective 'something' may be the lipoproteins. Among the Ashkenazi centenarians, about 80 percent had lipoprotein molecules 30 percent larger than the control group. Large lipoproteins are associated with less cardiovascular disease, less hypertension, and reduced rates of metabolic syndrome[68].

But the lipoproteins are just one factor among many. Reaching 100 is dependent on many other factors as well. It should be remembered that often longevity and good health do not always go together. Longevity is possible despite presence of one or more chronic disease.

The Genetic Secrets

The genetic studies in human centenarians may provide us an understanding of longevity in man. There is a tendency toward longevity clusters in families. In many centenarians' families, longevity appears to be a dominant trait, as many of their members live past 100. One in 10,000 people alive today do have longevity genes. The centenarians, in addition to being free of the negative genetic variations common in other human beings, also have some positive mutations that increase the possibility of longer life span. There appears to be a common mutation on chromosome 4 among centenarians.

The genetic studies reveal that certain subtle variations can cause changes in the way the gene works. Centenarians are a diverse group, so identifying shared traits having impact on longevity is not an easy task. In general, we all have the same genes, but vary from each other in SNPs or single nucleotide polymorphisms. The vast majority of these SNPs have no impact on longevity. But a few of them might increase the likelihood of high cholesterol, cardiovascular disease, or Alzheimer's disease. Negative mutations can accumulate in the course of evolution, as long as they do not affect fertility or life span during an organism's reproductive years.

IMPORTANCE OF RELAXATION AND SLEEP

In worms, the lifespan is essentially regulated by a hibernation cycle. When the worms enter hibernation, they are shutting themselves down. For humans, the closest thing to hibernation   is sleep, which is regulated by the nervous system. The persons living long lives perhaps do something very different from the rest while they sleep. Their bodies relax, doing something close to hibernation. Their bodies rejuvenate. There is, perhaps, certain genetic control that links hormonal signals regulating sleep and insulin signaling to longevity.

The studies prove that the centenarians may differ in body types, but all of them are positive people. They have stayed mostly healthy during their lives. There appears to be a hormonal state that is consistent with well-being and living a long time. It might be possible that a peptide hormone like insulin triggers high-level responses or the sorts of things that signal satiety.

Psychosocial factors like believing in God, having a social position, or simply owning a pet have been linked to longer life. These things point to some longevity pathways activated through neuronal hormones. These hormones may in turn be regulated by the level of satisfaction one finds in daily living.

PART FIVE

<u>FACTSHEET FOR LONGEVITY</u>

CHAPTER THIRTEEN

WHERE DO WE STAND?
Futuristic Visions of Longevity

WE, THE LIVING

Enthusiasm for living is the driving force behind the desire to live a long life. Also, it is the force behind working for the life extension. Not many people can believe in the possible life extension. They do not imagine potential for rejuvenation and perpetual youth; their mind is set by the age-old prejudices and fixations. But the survival instinct is winning over the obstacles and exciting changes are taking place in the scientific world of gerontology, biotechnology, and nano-biology. These hold immense promise as far as slowing the ageing and prolonging lifespan are concerned.

Despite widespread apathy and ignorance of science in our society, there has come awareness for health and fitness. People are looking forward for meaningful therapies, which can protect and preserve life. There is an increased awareness for fitness, longer life and lasting health.

It is quite reasonable to take the stock of the things, where do we stand? What lies in the store in near and far future? This exercise will guide us in warding off unreasonable expectations from the ageing research. At the same time, it will help in consolidating our issues on longevity.

IDEOLOGICAL DICHOTOMY
IN SCIENTIFIC CIRCLES

The optimism is infectious, but the pessimism is fatal. There prevails confusion in the sphere of science regarding the future of lifespan and longevity. The undue elation amounting to euphoria is unwanted as much as the despair, which mars the drive for scientific research.

• <u>Pessimistic Attitude in Scientific Circles</u>: **A number of** demographers predict that human lifespan will not increase any further and may even start to decline. The health of the adult generation is already declining. There is increasing disability afflicting adults below age 60. Obesity, diabetes, high blood pressure and heart disease are on the rise and curtail the visions of a healthier future. The drop in lifespan has already happened in some countries because of HIV/AIDS, and very recently because of COVID-19 pandemic. But no population is free from the threats of viral pandemics. In fact, future infections are likely to be fulminant and resistant to treatment. As they say, 'the human population is becoming like a dense forest with a lot of dry wood ready to burn'. The overall picture seems dismal.

• <u>Optimistic Attitude in Scientific Circles</u>: The assumption that life in future will be worse than what is today does not hold to be real in light of the progress in human knowledge and technology. There is a good reason that progress in knowledge and technology will go on. In the coming future we will win over the present obstacles. The whole new generation of futurist visionaries, believe that it will be possible to maintain human health at a youthful level for many extra decades by healthy living, employing new methods of anti-ageing medicine and rejuvenation science. For the first time in human history, we have come close to understanding human ageing and possible ways to slow it down.

THE MEANING OF LIFE EXTENSION

The Life extension stands for an increase in the maximum lifespan beyond the current maximum lifespan for humans. For those who regard ageing as a disease, therapeutic methods to extend maximum lifespan are anti-aging medicine.

It was in 1970, the American Ageing Association was formed under the initiative of Denham Harman, the originator of the free radical theory of ageing. The bestselling book, 'Life Extension' by Durk Pearson and Sandy Shaw popularized the phrase. The book dealt largely with antioxidant supplements. In 1980, the writer of the book 'The Life Extension Revolution', Saul Kent created the Life Extension Foundation, a non-profit organization. The Life Extension Foundation later established, the Alcor Life Extension Foundation, the largest cryonics organization.

In 1993 the American Academy of Anti-Ageing Medicine (A4M) was formed to create an anti-ageing medical specialty distinct from geriatrics. The most recent development in life extension has been the work of bio-gerontologist Aubrey de Grey. He proposes that damage to macromolecules, cells, tissues and organs can be repaired by advanced nano-biotechnology.

FUTURE POSSIBILITIES OF LIFE EXTENSION

It is true that we are far from fully understanding the biological principles of life. Yet, with our rapidly increasing knowledge of the human genome, and biochemical processes and pathways of metabolism, we are quickly beginning to understand ageing. Many scientists believe that soon we may be able to utilize the experience from lab researches for slowing the ageing process.

The visionaries see the life extension program going through three steps -

Step One: Taking advantage of the existing knowledge for slowing ageing, like caloric restriction with adequate nutrition (CRAN),

<u>Step Two</u>: Utilizing the advances in genetics and biotechnology, and

<u>Step Three</u>: Using the future nanotechnology and artificial intelligence revolution, which may have the potential to allow us to repair the mutations and other defects due to ageing at molecular and cellular levels.

THE VISIONS OF FUTURE:
PURSUING END OF AGEING:

The way to cure ageing is to rejuvenate tissues; not just to slow down their deterioration, i.e., slowing ageing. Thus, the futuristic goal is not only to slow ageing, but to achieve rejuvenation and state of non-ageing.

There are seven major types of damage that actually accumulate with age.

- First of all, there is cell loss. Certain tissues, like heart and brain, lose cells with ageing and these cells are not naturally replaced. The stem cell therapy can be used to restore the number of cells in these tissues.
- Second is, mutations in chromosomes. These mutations cause cancer and can affect the life span. The targeted gene therapy can be used to delete the telomere elongation genes in particular tissues at risk of developing cancer.
- Third is, the mitochondrial mutations. The insertional gene therapy can introduce modified versions of the 13 protein-coding mitochondrial genes into nuclear DNA. This will prevent accumulation of mutations in the mitochondrial DNA from affecting us as we age.
- Fourth is, the problem of senescent cells. Immune therapy can be used to destroy senescent cells.
- Fifth is, extracellular cross-linking. It can be possible to design drugs that can break the cross links between

long-lived molecules in the extra-cellular matrix, such as collagen and elastin.

- Sixth is, extra cellular junk, or garbage. This is most important in Alzheimer's disease and like. There is needed a therapy which can, not only, slow down the accumulation and but get rid of it as well. The insertional gene therapy can help by introducing bacterial or fungal genes that can break down damaging accumulated chemicals and proteins. Those to be tackled will include oxidized cholesterol that causes atherosclerosis, bis-retinoid N-retinyl-N-retinylidene ethanolamine (A2E) that is responsible for macular degeneration, and malformed proteins in the brain thought to be responsible for Alzheimer's, Parkinson's, and other neurodegenerative diseases.

- Finally, the seventh point is, to keep alive or preserved till the technology is practically available. Until molecular repair technologies are available, good health practices, supplements and organ transplantation, and cryopreservation after death are our best hope.

THE STEM CELL REVOLUTION

The regenerative properties of organs are tied to the behavior of stem cells. Stem cells are undifferentiated cells that can self-renew and differentiate into specialized cells of the organ or tissue in which they are found. They are responsible for maintaining and repairing the tissue or organ. But as the body ages, the molecules that regulate stem cells eventually change and inhibit their regenerative properties.

Enter the final decade of last Century; everybody started talking of stem cells. No doubt, stem cell technology holds potential to cure diseases, provide organs for transplantation, and above all, find ways to retard or even reverse ageing process.

The scientists have been developing a hydrogel, a polymer-based matrix for directing stem cell growth. The research could potentially lead to treatments for degenerative diseases like muscular dystrophy and therapies for other diseases involving the brain or circulatory system.

THE MIRAGE OF

21st CENTURY

Many experts believe that soon we will be adding more than a year to human life expectancy every year. In a decade, we may be able to stop ageing in mice, which shares 99 percent of our genetic code. The results may be applicable to humans in near future. These results will help in revitalizing our health and expanding our intelligence and capability. There will be profound changes in every facet of our lives, from our health and longevity to our economy and society. The basic concepts of life like human lifespan, who we are and what it means to be human are in for change.

THE BIOTECHOLOGY
REVOLUTION

Scientific strategies are emerging for overcoming disease and ageing processes. The backbone of the advancements is the information about the genome. With help of genetics and gene technology, the gene expressions can be controlled. Soon, changing the genes themselves may become possible. We are already using gene technology in various fields. By using recombinant technology, various pharmaceutical drugs like insulin are being manufactured. In the near future, scientists will be able to re-grow cells and tissues to produce a whole organ which can be used for transplantation.

These advances will revolutionize the rejuvenation medicine. The nanotechnology in alliance with advanced biology, nano-biotechnology, will help in designing drugs to act precisely at the molecular level.

VISIONS APART, WHERE DO WE STAND?

The visionaries walk in the time machine, often without feet on a firm ground. Visions of future are okay, but we should realize where do we stand today? Right now, neither we have the knowledge; nor the tools to live forever. If gerontological science and life extension technologies fail to show any further real advancement, the answer will be no to halting or reversing ageing. But we understand the process of ageing. We do have the means to slow ageing and prevent and satisfactorily treat various diseases and disorders. But there are no real and reliable technologies to indefinitely extend human life.

But the past is not always a consistent guide to the future. Also, the future cannot be taken for granted. However certain it may seem; the unpredictability remains and can mar visions of future. The human ability to take command of the course of life and death is controversial. But we have the ability to broaden our horizons, which is the most unique and desirable attribute of our species.

SOCIO-ECONOMIC EFFECTS OF LONGER LIVES

Early in the demographic cycle, the birth rates and death rates were both extremely high. As the societies advanced, nutrition, sanitation, and medicine all served to lower the death rate. The falling death rates accompanied by still high birth rates led to large population sizes. But in the last few decades the birth rate has also dropped sharply, especially in the developed countries. This demographic trend is spreading from Europe, Japan, and North America to the rest of the world.

The UN Population Division expects that the populations of Italy, Germany and Spain, most other European nations, and Japan will decrease over the next 50 years, despite the fact that there is appreciable increase in the life expectancy in these countries. At the other extreme are the fastest growing populations, with relatively low life expectancies, in countries like China, India, Pakistan, Bangladesh and Nigeria.

But taken together the birth rate worldwide is falling and the world population is growing at roughly 1 percent, much slower than in earlier times. In 2000, world population stood at 6 billion people, and in 2050, will be somewhere between 8 billion and 11 billion. The overall world population will level up and begin to drop. These projections, do not take into account, disease epidemics, natural calamities and killer technologies that can radically alter the prospect for mankind.

In this perspective, the impact of increased longevity on population is likely to be small. Further, it will not be instant, but gradual. Those, who are already of advanced age, are unlikely to benefit much from technology that can slow or halt ageing. The middle aged and young will benefit most.

SOCIO-POLITICAL CONFUSION AND HINDERANCES

The most important hindrance is public confusion about meaning and credibility of anti-ageing research. There is a group of people, which believes that anti-ageing interventions are neither possible nor desirable. They consider anti-ageing medicine as tampering with nature, which is both immoral and futile. There is a prevalent fatalism that nothing can be done to cure ageing. Here is required public education about the research efforts being done throughout the world.

A VISION CALLED IMMORTALITY

Immortality or eternal life is the concept of living for a potentially infinite length of time. Throughout history, humans have had the desire to live forever. The ideas of immortality exist since time immemorial. There are numerous symbols representing immortality and it has existed in mythological tales. The modern sci-fi writers have also woven immortal worlds in their fiction.

In more recent times, people have had their dead bodies cryo-preserved in the hope that advances in medical science will allow them to be unfrozen, cured, and restored to life at some point in the future.

There are three main causes of death: ageing, disease and trauma. The hardest cause of death to overcome is trauma. In the postulated future world where ageing will be correctable and diseases will be triumphed over, a trauma would still kill, unless the technology advances to such extent that a body can heal itself from a severe trauma (technological immortality), as it heals for the smaller ones.

An interesting possibility involves uploading the mind like a computer software on to a new human-body-form generated by cloning, or simply uploading human consciousness onto a computer system, and surviving in a virtual environment. Quantum immortality is the name for this kind of speculation.

The important aspects of current practical scientific thinking about immortality are human cloning, cryonics, and nanotechnology. These projections lead us to notions of an unending existence.

CHAPTER FOURTEEN

FROZEN LIFE, WARM DREAMS
Cryonics and Beyond

THE SUSPENDED LIFE:
CRYOFREEZING FOR FUTURE

Cryonics is the practice of freezing a body immediately after clinical death with the aim of enabling eventual revival in the remote future (Fig 25). The cryonics is, thus, a speculative life support technology that seeks to preserve human life in a state that will be viable and treatable by future medicine[69]. The cryopreservation which is based on a more sophisticated understanding of death called 'information-theoretic death', offers a bridge to the life in future[70].

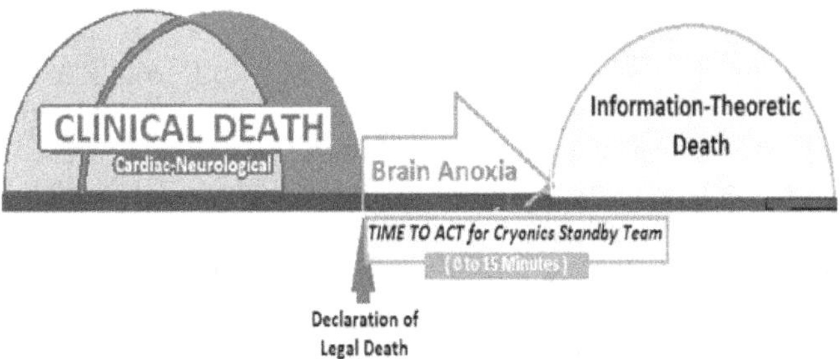

**Figure 25: Concepts for Cryonics -
Clinical-Legal and Information-Theoretic Death**

The current medical and legal definition of death is based on the cardiac arrest and the cessation of electrical activity in the cerebral cortex. Whereas, a person is dead according to the information theoretic criterion if the memories, personality, hopes, dreams, etc. have been destroyed in the information theoretic sense, and the structures in the brain that encode memory and personality have been so disrupted that it is no longer possible to recover them. The information-theoretic death is 'absolutely irreversible death' and the destruction of the brain has occurred to such an extent that any information it may have ever held is irrevocably lost for all eternity.

Further, the cryo-preserved bodies are not irreversibly dead as per the information-theoretic definition of death. They are kept indefinitely preserved in a thermos-type container filled with liquid nitrogen until the cryo-preservation damage would be possibly reversed at some time in future when the advanced state of science and technology will allow the cause of the fatal disease to be cured and repair the damage to the body because of the ageing process.

CRYOPRESERVATION IN ACTION
FREEZING LIFE FOR FURURE

The cryopreservation process should start immediately after clinical-legal death is declared as organs remain biologically alive for some time, and vitrification, particularly of the brain, is possible. The clinical-legal death declaration indicates that there is nothing more can be done by the medical personnel to save the patient. Of course, the declaration of death does not mean that life has suddenly ended - death is not a sudden event but a gradual process. The Stand-by Cryonics Team acts immediately, to minimize ischemic and reperfusion injury by beginning cardiopulmonary support and cooling as soon as possible after pronouncement of death (Fig 26), as the body is suitable for cryopreservation or the preservation of the brain for a short time only.

The body is cooled to just above 0°C and the blood is replaced with a preservant and a solution is injected to stop ice crystals formation in organs and tissues. Thereafter, the body is further cooled gradually to -130°C and the anti-freeze compounds are injected to stop damage to the cells. The finally the body is placed in a container which is lowered into a tank of liquid nitrogen at -196°C.

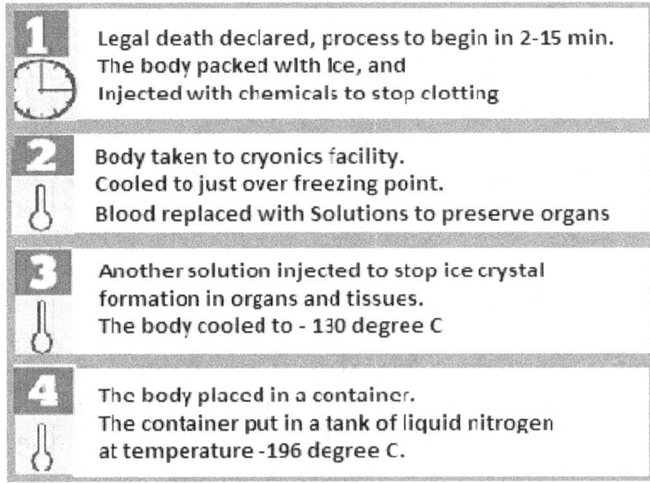

Figure 26: Cryopreservation in action

Alternatively, the head with brain inside is cryopreserved in liquid nitrogen at -196°C, contained in the Dewar flask, an insulated container which consumes no electric power. Newer forms of cryonics use a process called vitrification. The vitrification employs low temperatures and cryoprotectants to turn tissue into a glass-like state where decay is extremely slow. It is also possible to develop hybrid procedures involving elements of both cryonics and chemical brain preservation.

HEAD (NEURO-) Vs. WHOLE-BODY CROPRESERVATION

During the 1980s, the cryonics corporations shifted emphasis from whole body to 'neuro-preservation' (i.e. head-only cryopreservation), with the assumption that the rest of the body could be regrown and reconstructed in future by nanobiotechnology. The main goal now is to preserve the information contained in the structure of the brain, on which memory and personal identity depend, and the available scientific and medical evidence suggests that the mechanical structure of the brain called connectome, is wholly responsible for personal identity and memories. The chemical brain preservation, viewed as a life-saving medical procedure, allows the brain to be preserved for a long period and in the future, the information in a chemically preserved brain may be able to be decoded and emulated in a computer. The main limitation of current cryonics is the uncertainty whether the information in the brain is truly preserved, though there is indirect evidence that cryonics preserves the information in the brain which could be recovered.

The hypothesis of chemical brain preservation as life extension was proposed by Drexler in 1987 and Olson in 1988[71]. The brain is completely responsible for the mind and the identity is defined by anatomy: that is, brain connectivity. Our memories and personalities are captured in the synaptic and dendritic connections in the brain, referred to as the connectome. The information theory of death and understanding of the connectome imply that death does not occur until the information in the connectome is irreversibly lost. In the distant future, technology may advance to the state where the information of an individual's brain design can be extracted from the preserved brain and the complete connectome to be obtained from preserved brains, the whole brain emulation (WBE)[72].

Knowledge of the connectome should allow for a complete emulation of brain function, and the technologies for mapping the connectome and for WBE have been advancing rapidly. The development of WBE and the computer technology to implement it is now an initiative of the European Union known as the Human Brain Project, which aims to develop a complete emulation of a mouse brain and later that for the human brain. The Human Brain

Project aims to scan and upload a significant portion of the human brain.

Some critics, and some cryonicists, question this emphasis on the brain. Because during neuro-preservation, the information about the body's phenotype will be lost. Also, the body is personal memorabilia of life-history. But the lower costs and better brain preservation may justify preserving only the brain.

HUMAN BRAIN PROJECT

Decoding the human brain may be one of the most fascinating scientific challenges in the 21st century. The Human Brain Project (HBP) targets the reconstruction of the brain's multi-scale organization by using medical data, data analytics and simulation experiments[73].

The HBP, based in Geneva, was started in 2013 under European Commission and Future and Emerging Technologies flagship. The primary objective of the HBP is to create an Information and Communication Technology (ICT) based research base for brain research, cognitive neuroscience, and brain-inspired computing, for researchers world-wide. The HBP also undertakes targeted research and theoretical studies to explore brain structure and function in humans, rodents and other species.

There are six ICT research platforms related to the HBP project - Neuro-informatics (access to shared brain data), Brain Simulation (replication of brain architecture and activity on computers), High Performance Analytics (providing required computing and analytics capabilities), Medical Informatics (access to patient data and identification of disease signatures), Neuromorphic Computing (development of brain-inspired computing) and Neurorobotics (use of robots to test brain simulations). The usefulness of WBE and HBP for the cryonics related neuro-preservation and restoration later can be only a hypothetical conjecture at present.

CRYONICS TODAY:
THE FACTSHEET

Over 350 people worldwide have had their bodies preserved in cryogenic chambers after death in the hope to be revived in distant future. The experts at the Cryonics Institute (CI), Michigan have claimed that cryonically bringing someone back to life should definitely be doable in 100 years or sooner. The CI has about 160 patients frozen in specialised tanks of liquid nitrogen at its headquarters; and has almost 2,000 people signed up to be frozen later when they die. Two main US cryonics organisations are Alcor at Arizona, and the CI at Michigan. A Russian body KrioRus and Alcor's European laboratory in Portugal are the two facilities outside the US to offer the service. Aside from Trans Time, the other three cryonics organizations in the world which are storing human patients in liquid nitrogen are the Alcor Life Extension Foundation (founded in 1972 by Fred and Linda Chamberlain), the Cryonics Institute (founded in 1976 by Robert Ettinger), and KrioRus (located near Moscow in Russia, founded in 2006). It is being claimed that cryonics may replace traditional burials and cremations in the next few decades, leading to Cryo-Parlours in place of Funeral Parlours.

FUTURISTIC VISIONS OF LONGEVITY:
THE EXPONENTIAL LIFESPAN

Anti-ageing and Rejuvenation Science

In the current times, there is an increased awareness for fitness and health, and enthusiasm for living a long life. The latter is winning over the prejudices, fixations and obstacles, and exciting changes are taking place in the scientific world of gerontology, biotechnology and nanobiology which hold immense promise for slowing the ageing and prolonging lifespan. The healthy ageing puts forth three options before us. One, we can try to improve metabolism so that it generates less harmful by-products as by CR; two, we can clean up these by-products; and three, deal with the consequences of the accumulation of damage over time.

Where do we stand on the issue of prolonging lifespan and what lies in store for us in the near and far future? What are the expectations from the ageing research and the projections and fallouts? The futurist visionaries believe that it will be possible to maintain human health at a youthful level for many extra decades by healthy living, employing new methods of anti-ageing medicine and rejuvenation science to retard and probably reverse the ageing. Since ageing is consequence of the damage accumulation, repair of the damage forms the basis of rejuvenation, the reversal of ageing and prevention of degenerative and age-related diseases. The regenerative therapies aim to remove, repair, replace or render harmless the accumulated cellular and molecular damage and restore the normal functioning of the tissues and essential biomolecules (Fig 27).

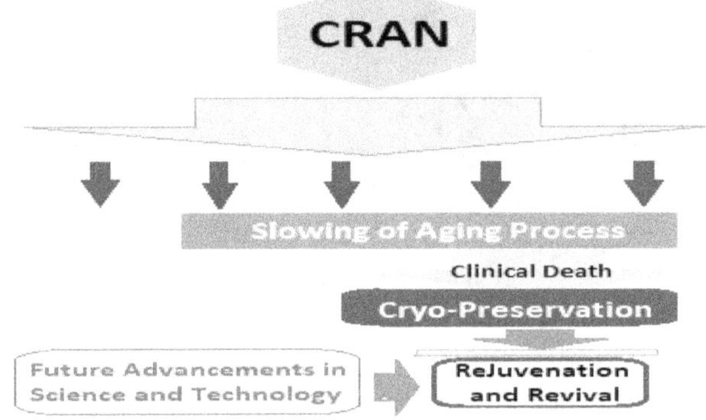

Figure 27: The Future Projections for Exponential Longevity, Damage repair, Rejuvenation and Revival

Visions for Exponential Life Extension

The Life extension stands for an increase in the maximum lifespan beyond the current maximum lifespan for humans, and the exponential life extension can be defined as increase in life expectancy and life span by 50 per cent or more. For those who regard ageing as a disease, therapeutic methods to extend maximum lifespan are anti-ageing medicine. The recent development in life extension is the vision that the damage to macromolecules, cells, tissues and organs can be repaired by advanced nanobiotechnology. As we understand the biological principles of life and ageing process, and able to utilize the experimental research, the life extension program (LEP) can be seen as a plausible step in near future. The LEP is projected to go through three steps - Step One: Taking advantage of the existing knowledge for slowing ageing through interventions like CR; Step Two: Utilizing the advances in genetic engineering and biotechnology; and Step Three: Using the future nanotechnology and artificial intelligence revolution to repair mutations and other defects due to ageing at molecular and cellular levels (Fig 28).

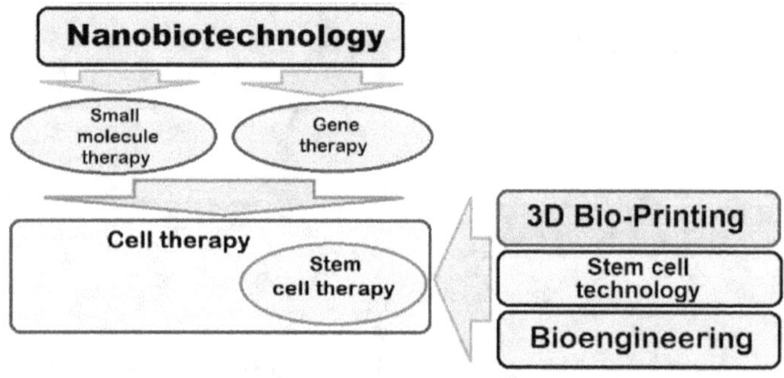

Figure 28: LEP through advanced future technologies - Genetic engineering, Nanobiotechnology and Stem cell technology.

The way to cure ageing is to rejuvenate tissues, not just to retard ageing. The futuristic goal, thus, is to achieve rejuvenation and the state of non-ageing.

HISTORY AND DEVEOPMENT
CRYONICS SCIENCE

Benjamin Franklin suggested, long back in 1773, that it might be possible to preserve human life in a suspended state for centuries. In 1962, Robert Ettinger proposed in his book, 'The Prospect of Immortality', that freezing people may be a way to reach future medical technology. He argued that the early stages of clinical death may be reversible in the future and freezing recently deceased people may be a way to save lives. With this understanding, began the modern era of cryonics. Almost simultaneously, Evan Cooper also suggested and worked on the same idea and founded the Life Extension Society in 1965 to promote freezing people after clinical death.

The word, cryonics, was coined in 1965 by Karl Werner. The cryonics societies were founded in New York, Michigan, and California. In 1976, the Cryonics Institute, a cryonics service organization was founded by Robert Ettinger. The first person successfully frozen with intent of future revival was a lung cancer patient, Dr James Bedford, in January 1967, who died at age of 74.

The largest cryonics organization today is the Alcor Society for Solid State Hypothermia (ASSSH), now renamed the Alcor Life Extension Foundation. It was proved that cardiac and pulmonary resuscitation (CPR) and certain medications applied immediately after cardiac arrest, followed by cardiopulmonary bypass and thoracic surgery for access to major blood vessels, could greatly reduce ischemic injury in cryonics patients. There evolved, thus, the cryonics procedure, called 'Standby', in which a stabilization team stands by to institute life support procedures at the bedside of a cryonics patient as soon as possible after the clinical death is announced.

Cryonics received new support in the 1980s when there evolved the new field of molecular nanotechnology. Advocates for cryonics saw the nascent field of nanotechnology as vindication of, their long-held view that molecular repair of injured tissue was theoretically possible. In the 1990s the damaging effects of freezing were revealed in detail. There developed the trend to use higher concentrations of glycerol, a cryo-protectant to prevent freezing injury. In 2001 Alcor began using vitrification in an attempt to prevent ice formation during initiation of cryopreservation.

In 2005 Alcor began applying vitrification treatment to the whole body. At the same time, the Cryonics Institute began using a new procedure in which the head is vitrified while still attached to the body, which is frozen without any cryoprotectant. Alcor currently maintains about 70 cryonics patients in Scottsdale, Arizona and the Cryonics Institute has about the same number of cryonics patients in its Clinton Township, Michigan facility. Apart from the cryonics service providers in the United States, there are various support groups in Europe, Canada, Australia, and the United Kingdom.

THE CRYONICS, AS TODAY

Cryonics is not a widespread medical practice. Its support is based on controversial projections of future technologies and of their ability to enable molecular-level repair of tissues and organs. The cryonics is different from mummification, which simply stands for the preservation of the dead body.

Viruses, bacteria, sperm/eggs, embryos at early stages of development, insects, and even small animals, such as small frogs and fish, have been cryo-frozen, and preserved for an indefinite time and then thawed and returned to a living state. An organism put in liquid nitrogen, whether frozen or vitrified, is said to be cryo-preserved. Barring social disruptions, cryonicists believe that a perfectly vitrified person can be expected to remain physically viable for about 30,000 years, after which the damage due to cosmic rays may be irreparable.

But the justification for the actual practice of cryonics is unclear, given the primitive state of preservation technology. It may appear like keeping mummies in pyramids. The advocates, however, say that even a slim chance of revival is better than no chance. In the future, they speculate, medical science is likely to conquer ageing and death, and accomplish molecular-level tissue repair leading to revival. Thus, if one could preserve one's body or at least the brain and some tissues for another hundred years, they conjure, one might well be resuscitated and able to live indefinitely long. While technology today cannot do revival, it can well preserve the body and detailed structure of the brain.

A group of cryonicists visualizes that if technology is developed that allows mind transfer, revival of the frozen brain might not even be required. The possibility that body and brain of a person could be cloned from the preserved tissues and then the mind of the person could be uploaded into the new substrate (the cloned brain), like a computer software.

DEALING WITH
THE ICE FORMATION

The large animals or organs cannot be safely frozen because removing heat from thick tissues by natural thermo-conductivity becomes so slow that ice microcrystals grow big enough to damage cell organelle and membranes leading to any future repair impossible. But this problem has been overcome by the improvements in cryopreservation technology, including new cryo-protectants and new cryo-protectant mixtures, which greatly improve the feasibility of vitrification and result in the near-elimination of ice crystal formation in the brain and other organs.

Vitrification preserves tissue in a glassy rather than frozen state. Further, the solutions used for vitrification are stable enough to avoid crystallization even when a vitrified brain is warmed up. This has recently allowed brains to be vitrified, warmed back up, and examined for ice damage using light and electron microscopy. No ice crystal damage was found. However, if the circulation of the brain is compromised, protective chemicals may not be able to reach all parts of the brain, and freezing may occur either during cooling or during re-warming.

CRYOPRESERVATION:
THE FINANCIAL ISSUES

The biggest drawback of the cryo-preservation is its cost. The most cost-effective means of storing a cryo-preserved person is in liquid nitrogen. But fracturing of the brain occurs, during the process, as a result of thermal stresses that develop when cooling from −130°C to −196°C (the temperature of liquid nitrogen).

The fracture-free vitrification would require expensive storage at a temperature significantly below the glass transition temperature of about −125°C, but high enough to avoid fracturing (−130°C is about right). Current vitrification method is far superior to traditional glycerol-based freezing. Further research and advancements are taking place.

Cryopreservation arrangements can be expensive, currently ranging from $28,000 at the Cryonics Institute to $150,000 at Alcor and the American Cryonics Society. Further, the cryopreserved people are to be maintained for an indefinite period. But, all in all, cryonics is actually quite affordable for many in the industrialized world if they find it attractive and endorse it.

Even assuming perfect cryopreservation techniques, many cryonicists would still regard eventual revival as a long shot. In addition to many technical hurdles that remain, the likelihood of obtaining a good cryopreservation is not very high because of logistical problems. The likelihood of the continuity of cryonics organizations as businesses, and the threat of legislative interference in the practice, do not help the odds either. Most cryonicists, however, regard their cryopreservation arrangements as something better than no chance at all and still a rational gamble to take.

CRYONICS:
FICTION AND FACTS

Cryonics is often seen in sci-fi as a means to transport a character from the past into the future. In addition to accomplishing whatever the character's primary task is in the future, he or she must cope with the strangeness of a new world. The movie, 'Demolition Man', features two characters, a police officer and villain, who are frozen in the late 20th century. They are unfrozen forty years later where they must learn the strange ways in which the new world works.

While, most trans-humanists are quite convinced that life extension will be possible, most agree that it will take several decades or even centuries before non-ageing or immortality becomes actually possible. In the meantime, one can die from accidents or disease, regardless of how healthy the lifestyle is. The only answer to this problem is cryo-preservation. Thus, on untimely death, one's body can be preserved until medical techniques have been developed to the extent to revive, repair and cure.

Recapitulating the state of affairs, as is today, there is little to lose by choosing cryo-preservation. Either it will work and restoration methods will be developed and used in the far future, or it will not. So, the rational choice apparently is to use cryonics, even if success seems improbable at this point of time.

CHAPTER FIFTEEN
DARK-SIDE OF LIFE EXTENSION:
Tithonus Option, Life on Support, Etc.

THE FEARS ASSOCIATED WITH EXTENDED LIFE

Future technology appears to offer us visions that rival the dreams of myth and legend. According to the Clarke's Law - 'any sufficiently advanced technology is indistinguishable from magic.' One of these dreams is that of extended life. It appears that with the advancements in medical science, genetics, biotechnology, coupled with those in nanotechnology, a true extension of human lifespan will come in the near future. However, it may come at a price.

The Tithonus Option

There is a fear that the anti-ageing technology may present us with the extended lifespan but limited improvement in quality of life. The nightmare, that we will live longer but in bad health and mental deterioration, has been named the Tithonus option - immortal life with sub-functional brain or eternal dementia[74].

<u>The Story of Tithonus:</u> Tithonus, a mortal, fell in love with Eos, the goddess of the dawn in Greek mythology. The goddess, Eos, knowing that the mortal, Tithonus was destined to age and die, begged Zeus, the supreme god of ancient Greek mythology and counterpart of Roman god Jupiter, to grant her lover an immortal life. Zeus, the jealous god, granted the wish but not the eternal youth. With passing time, Tithonus aged, becoming increasingly debilitated and demented, eventually driving Eos to distraction. In despair, she turned Tithonus into a grasshopper. In Greek mythology, the grasshopper is immortal.

There are several foreseeable outcomes from the anti-ageing technology. Today, the majority of people living in the developed countries can expect to live well into their seventies. Even so, the final years are usually marked by impaired health and impaired cognitive functions. Here, three possible futuristic outcomes may seem probable: The first, we will live and die as we do today and there may accrue no benefit of ageing research. The second possibility, called the Tithonus option, is that the technology will give extended lifespan but will not be able to reduce prevalence of cognitive impairment and debility. The third possible outcome is that technology will be able to repair the damage done with age to our body tissues and organs including neurons, thus granting us longevity with good quality of life.

<u>The Failure of Success</u>: People now a days are increasingly live to old age for many reasons including improved social standards, preventative measures for conditions like infectious diseases and better access to medical care for diseases like cardiovascular disease and cancer. A far proportion of population reach old age after various medical procedures and interventions, and dependent on various medications. As a consequence, older adults are increasingly seen in hospitals and by healthcare professionals. This phenomenon has been called 'the failure of success' by Gruenberg where success in preventing death has led to more prevalent morbidity and chronic illness[75].

<u>COVID-19 Pandemic and Healthcare</u>: Generally, we find medical decision-making favours more investigation, active treatment, and intervention in the acutely ill patients, and more so in elderly patients with associated chronic diseases. During the present COVID-19, the approach has become more pragmatic for judicious use of scarce resources. In this light, physicians in Italy and elsewhere

were falling to an approach that focuses on the priorities in healthcare especially those in need of intensive care[76].

With the healthcare becoming dehumanized, the doctors were not abandoning the elderly or making them more disadvantaged, they ensured that care was not compromised in the unavailing quest for a longer life.

It remains to be seen whether in a post-COVID-19 era, we will return to our pursuit of longevity and immortality, with the Tithonism resurrected[77].

The Senile Brain Disease

The age-specific prevalence of serious mental disorders rises rapidly in the last decades of life. As the general population is aging, so prevalence of SBD is increasing. Clinical diagnosis of senile dementia is common, but simultaneously, there exist a large number of asymptomatic silent cases. The incidence of SBD soars between age 70 and age 80, begin to fall off after age 80.

There are no means of diagnosing senile plaques, which can make an early diagnosis of SBD. By the time, diagnosis of SBD is made, the disease may be in an advanced stage. The new evidence about aluminium deposits in the senile plaques suggests the possibility that a non-invasive test may be developed to ascertain the presence of such deposits.

The only clinical differences between senile and presenile dementia of the Alzheimer type relate to age of onset and rapidity of course, the presenile variety showing a more fulminant progression.

Life on Support Systems

In the intensive care units, it is commonly seen that for the critically ill patients, more and more invasive procedures are performed to save the life and more and more of the vital functions are taken over by bio-machines. The ventilator drives the respiration, intravenous fluids infusion and drugs provide the nutrition and support the vital functions. Gradually more mechanical devices including the ECMO (extracorporeal membrane oxygenation) or the heart and lung machine take over. The person is considered living till the brain function persists. It is an artificially prolonged life on support systems, amounting to a nightmare of proportion of the Tithonus option amounting to a long life, with zero quality of life.

Just consider the renal disease patients in whom the kidneys have totally failed, they are maintained on dialysis, since even a poor-quality-of-life is better than no life. Will we not fall in the same trap, finally reconciling ourselves to Tithonus option? People may regard it better than cryo-preservation in hope of a novel treatment in the remote future. Thus, the Tithonus option is feared. The optimistic scientists, though, think that the Tithonus Option is not a likely outcome for various reasons.

Seen from a common perspective, while the persons suffering from chronic diseases are getting their life extended by modern day treatment, they are also getting an extension of disease and disability. In future too, while genetic engineering and nanotechnology may help in extending the life significantly, it does not follow that future technology will be able to repair all wear-and-tear on the brain and body organs. If the future technology cannot repair all microscopic injuries, the Tithonus option will result.

THE FUTURE VISIONS AND THE GURSKY SOLUTION

Current patterns of death: The death rate increases exponentially because our bodies accumulate damage. The accumulated mutational load over time leads to errors in DNA leading to cancer. It takes years of accumulated mutations for cells to become cancerous.

The vascular disease is the result of narrowing of and plaque deposition in arteries because of the atherosclerosis process. The heart attack occurs when blood supply is interrupted to a part of heart. The stroke occurs when a clot breaks off from an arterial plaque and lodges in an artery supplying a part of brain. A stroke can also occur when an artery bursts in the brain, pouring out blood under pressure. The resulting blood clot damages brain tissue by a direct pressure effect. As such, the vascular disease represents an example of accumulated errors.

The accidental deaths follow a complex curve. Young people are more likely to die of accidents than those older. This is due to the higher prevalence of risk-taking behaviours. As the age increases, there comes awareness for safety. The elderly, too, are more likely to die because of accidents. Reduced balance and co-ordination, delayed response, muscular weakness, and osteoporosis put the elderly at greater risk of having an accident. In the elderly, accidental deaths show an exponential curve because, they are the result of accumulated damage.

The Gursky Solution: The diseases of accumulated damage are destined to be the primary causes of death in developed countries. Also, with development, in other countries too, the deaths from infectious diseases will reduce, emulating the patterns seen in developed countries.

The only possible escape from the diseases of accumulated damage, is developing advanced medical technologies capable of repairing the wear and tears in tissues, and mutational errors. This is called the Gursky solution, named after Ian McDonald's novel, 'The Days of Solomon Gursky'. In this sci-fi tale, the nano-tech inventions allow to ward-off disease processes and improve the human bodies.

The exponential death rates and increasing debility, with advancing age, go hand in hand. By solving one, the other can show a favourable trend. Thus, by decreasing cancer and accident deaths, we can look forward to reduce debility. Therefore, developing the anti-ageing technology will not lead to the Tithonus option but rather the Gursky solution.

EFFECTS OF EXTENDED LIFESPANS ON THE SOCIETY

The Vision of Life Extension

To stay alive is the basic human instinct. It is, also, a precondition for all other activities. Life-extension is the direct natural progression of curing diseases by treatment and preventing the effects of ageing. The human life is sacred and should be cherished and preserved.

The Fear of Social Burden

The extended life spans will definitely affect human society. It will bring positive effects on society of comprising of people with the wisdom of 150 years or more and the youthful vitality.

The issue of overpopulation should not be feared. In technologically advanced societies, couples tend to have fewer children, often below the replacement rate. By spread of benefits of technology, education, and women's rights, fertility rates will decline. As the UN population studies predict, over-population will be an unlikely fall-out of extended lifespan.

On the other hand, life extension will not place a burden on health care, as feared. The life extension, itself, is likely to be associated with good health and disability limitation. The older adults with extended life will be economically productive members of society.

Boring Long Life? Nope.

People on learning life extension projects, or sometimes, even scientists, convey the fear that living very long may be boring. But, feeling bored is a state of mind. The state is never permanent, it is a transient phase influenced by immediate situations. We discover new things, find something hidden in the things known for long and feeling of boredom passes away, replaced by the joy of excitement.

THE FUTURE
NON-AGEING WORLD

By eliminating a majority of age-related diseases and maintaining the vitality of the body for a very long time, we can look forward to achieving a significantly long lifespan of more than 1,000 years.

This estimation of future average life span of 1,000 years has been reached by considering the removal of age-related mortality from current statistics. Accidents and other such causes of death will still remain.

The anticipated problem of over-population apart, there will be other dangers. The people considered threats to the society at large, someone like Hitler and Stalin will remain in power much longer than they would if they faded away or died because of ageing. Criminals, too, would live longer like characters in cartoon films, continuing to pose a threat.

The delayed ageing will lead to various social changes. The age stratification in the society will disappear, and along with it, many of our current social mores. The new ideas and new possibilities will evolve.

PART SIX

<u>REALIZING THE DREAM</u>

CHAPTER SIXTEEN
THE HEALTHY LONGEVITY
Defeating the Ageing
177-186

CHAPTER SEVENTEEN
THE SUCCESSFUL AGEING:
Staying Alive and Well
187-193

CHAPTER SIXTEEN

THE HEALTHY LONGEVITY:
Defeating the Ageing

CHANGING OUR
PERCEPTION OF AGEING

The significant increase in average life expectancy is one of the major events of our times. This demographic change has led to a social rearrangement. This has also led to an overall changing pattern of the population and altered the resource utilization by population groups and generated new opportunities for older adults. But such rapid changes have left most of us living in the past with age-old prejudices both about ageing and elderly people. These outmoded beliefs are also embedded in the healthcare and social programs because the way we think about the older adults strongly influences the way in which we provide care for them.

Today, fewer than 25 percent of older adults experience any disability and fewer than 5 percent of them require bed-care. Intellectually, they work with zest and competence well beyond the traditional age of retirement. They combine an emotional maturity with wisdom that come with age. They are able to connect with their colleagues across age groups. The chronological age has lost its meaning as an index of individual capacity.

But many older adults need healthcare and other supports including emotional ad social one, like other age groups. This can only be provided suitably by abandoning the irrational prejudices.

IMPROVING HEALTH CARE
FOR OLDER ADULTS

It is important to commit to excellence in every field. The mediocrity has no place even in the care of older adults. For optimal health care for older adults, the following points should be considered –

• The overall intention is to help: To be of assistance to an older adult in need of relief from distress, guidance, or support. Like elsewhere, here too the patient needs an undivided attention.

• The second principle is working to increase the caregiver's perceptive capacity and patience. Perceive stress, if any and act accordingly.

• There should be a sense of conscious appreciation, respect, and reverence directed toward the older adults. The art of caring for the patient is also important.

TENNETS OF HEALTH CARE FOR OLDER ADULTS

The process of ageing is a continuum and spans throughout the life. It affects all older adults, though the rate of ageing varies widely. It is genetically programmed and modified by environmental influences. In the older adults, the spectrum of symptoms is broader; the manifestations of distress more subtle; and the improvement often less dramatic and slower to appear.

Because of the magnitude and associated complexity of medical, psychological, and social factors, the older adults require a clinical perspective that differ substantially from that for younger persons. Their healthcare should involve a holistic approach and take in account of not only physical and mental health, but also social and spiritual health (Fig 29). The older adults are more prone to suffer from deficiencies in these areas.

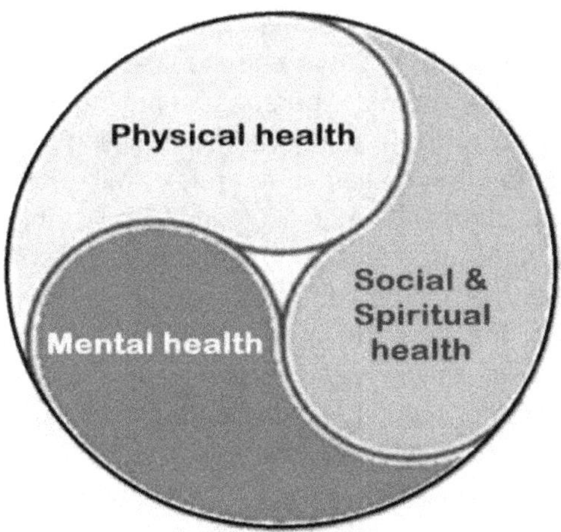

Figure 29: The social health and spiritual health are often neglected areas in older adults

Further, the increasing biological uniqueness of older persons as they age requires an individualized approach to their medical care. The medical interventions in older adults should aim to restore and maintain independent living and ability to function.

ENSURING ATOMOSPHERE THAT HEALS

• The attitudes of physicians and other healthcare personnel strongly influence the quality of care. The clinician's job is to reduce morbidity and improve function and quality of life. This is important because the presence of disease and the development of symptoms are not always closely related. In the older adults, eliminating the cause of distress may not be possible in many circumstances, so the focus lies in helping to relieve the distress itself. This care-oriented attitude is a bit different from the cure-oriented pre-set of mind.

• An attention to some specific environmental considerations can improve communication by facilitating sensory input to the older person and putting him or her at ease. Reducing the distance between sitting places, and encouraging the patients to relax will help. Office equipment should be practical and comfortable. Sitting down to talk is important. In fact, the importance of sitting is inversely proportional to the time available for the encounter: the less the time available, the greater the importance of sitting. Besides providing a common level for eye contact, sitting helps to neutralize the appearance of impatience and haste, which may magnify the hierarchic relationship (provider over patient), rather than establishing a partnership to solve problems.

• The biological age and chronological age are not same. Different individuals age differently. The physical ageing occurs in different organs systems at different rates, influenced by many factors. As we age, we become more unique and differentiated and less like one another. Further, because of this increasing biological variability with ageing, the clinical approach must be individualized.

AGEING RELATED CHANGES
Vs. DISEASE PROCESS

• Normal ageing in the absence of disease is a remarkably benign process. It involves a steady erosion of organ system reserves and homeostatic controls. The erosion may be evident only during periods of maximal exertion or stress. This structural and functional erosion leads to dysfunction and may reach a critical point during advanced age. Deviations from this ideal represent the effects of superimposed disease.

• Ageing also causes certain changes in body composition and in the structural elements of tissues. These changes have implications for nutritional planning, physical activity, and use of drugs.

• Because of the age-related physiological changes, diagnostic   investigation and treatment response are likely to be less than optimal.

• Another implication of ageing is the prospect of living with diminishing resources. The decline in functional reserve is compounded by losses of social status, income, family support, and self-esteem.

• The disease processes lead to reduced physical and mental capabilities, which are magnified by rapidly changing social expectations. The complexity of changing social expectations may be especially problematic for older adults. In addition, some older persons may be victims of changes in the physical environment. Some neighbourhoods, comfortable earlier may deteriorate into uncomfortable zones.

POTENTIALLY MODIFIABLE EFFECTS OF AGEING

The potential effects of ageing are variable and depend on Many factors. In general, they can be understood as following (Fig 30). A in the Figure represents the maximal possible potential performance for a given organ, such as the musculoskeletal or cardiovascular system. The slope B represents the maximum possible level of fitness, considering the decline only due to the age-related changes. The lower slope C represents a dis-functioning system due to disease and age-related changes.

The system always functions at some point between the slope B and slope C. The differences in slope B and slope C can be modified suitably by optimal lifestyle changes like dietary habits, physical activity, adopting healthy behavioral

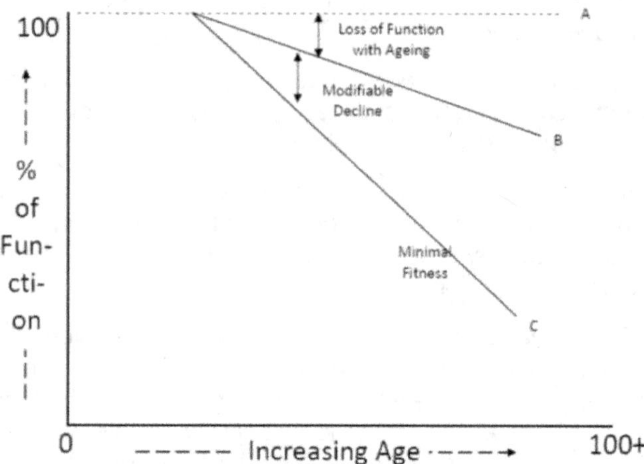

Figure 30: The effects of Ageing and Disease

habits (stopping smoking and drinking), a positive attitude; and optimal health care.

PRESENTATION OF DISEASE IN OLDER ADULTS

The major factors altering clinical presentation of disease in older adults are -

1. The under-reporting of illness: The older adults often under-report significant symptoms of illness. This may be due to personal attitudes and social isolation. On the other hand, the manifestations of disease may be dismissed as age-related changes, by the person himself or the family, or even the healthcare professionals. The depression can also limit the interaction in some older adults. Similarly, denial may be another reason for the underreporting. This may result from fear of economic, social, or functional consequences. Another important reason is the isolation,

which simply reduces the opportunity for receiving health care.

2. The changes in presentation of illness: The existence of multiple chronic diseases in some older adults may change the presenting symptoms and signs. Symptoms of one condition may either exacerbate or mask clinical features of the of another.

3. The altered response to illness: An older adult's perception of illness may be modified by attitudinal factors, social factors, and changes in the sensory organs. Manifestations of clinically important disease may be attenuated in those who are frail and disabled.

TREATMENT PRIORITIES IN OLDER ADULTS

Maximization of well-being, happiness, productivity, and creativity are the goals of healthcare in that order, for older adults. This goal of improving function may often be achieved without curing the underlying disease. The diagnostic tests may delay treatment and are often a futile exercise in older adults.

The fatalism and myth of constancy of one's lifespan affects the quality care and leads to neglect by self and others. Delaying the onset or progression of a chronic illness is as important as curing the underlying chronic disease. The functioning can often be improved without directly dealing with the underlying disease. For example, treatment of urinary incontinence does not depend on the cause of the bladder instability, which can be due to brain trauma, cerebrovascular accidents, or dementia caused by Alzheimer's disease.

The elderly patients often present with several chronic diseases, many of which are, often, irreversible.

Nevertheless, the discomfort or disability they produce may be substantially modified. Further, most of the disability experienced by older adults commonly results from diseases like atherosclerosis, diabetes, osteoarthritis, or chronic lung disease, which are complicated by the age-related physio-logical decline.

ADDING HEALTHY YEARS TO LATER LIFE

Today people, in general, are living longer. But many older adults suffer from various preventable health problems, which can be prevented or diminished.

The three Ps, Prevent, Protect and Plan, are important for optimal healthcare to reduce suffering and add healthy years to life in general -

• Preventive measures: Many older adults die because of influenza and pneumonia every year. Immunizations can reduce the incidence of hospitalization and death from these diseases. Many older adults knowingly skip their medication for diabetes, high blood pressure or heart disease. They are more likely to suffer from the complications. Accidents and falls at home or workplace can be prevented by measures like removing tripping hazards, replacing slippery floors and installing grab bars.

• Adopting healthy lifestyles: The older adults, who are physically active, should eat a healthy diet, resort to an exercise plan and practice healthy lifestyle and behaviours. A positive attitude and keeping the emotional stress at minimum are helpful. These simple factors will improve the QOL in general and health, in particular.

• Choosing a smoke-free life: The tobacco-related diseases kill millions of people worldwide. A good number of them are from the older adult groups. So, making the choice to stop smoking amounts to gaining healthy years of life. The studies tell us that soon after quitting smoking, the risk of heart disease, stroke and lung cancer.

STAYING HEALTHY
IN OLDER ADULTHOOD

In general, most of the older adults are quite health conscious. They understand that adopting healthy attitudes, active lifestyle and a balanced diet can help in staying healthy as they age. But, often the lack of motivation stands in the way.

The following points can help:

• Think right and eat right for healthy ageing: A positive attitude, eating well, exercising, and regular health check-ups are important. Nearly eighty percent of healthy ageing depends on diet, exercise, and attitude, and just twenty percent on the genes.

• Self-evaluation and assessment of health: A regular objective self-assessment of health, lifestyle and workup helps in the overall health management, including getting proper healthcare in time.

• Building on motivation: To stay healthy one must have a strong motivation. Lack of motivation is, often, the main obstacle, followed by lack of money. The main reasons for not getting health check-up may be the fear of discovering something awesome.

• Concern about callousness and cost of healthcare: Many of the older adults express some pessimism about the healthcare system as a whole. They find uncaring and callous healthcare professionals and paramedics who are prejudiced against the older adults. They fear that they will be denied the optimal care. Their main concern of the cost is often followed by the access and quality of healthcare.

OPTIMAL HEALTHCARE FOR OLDER ADULTS

The optimal healthcare for older adults necessitates a multifaceted approach incorporating collaboration of health, social welfare, and legal sectors. A strong political commitment and social action at community level like social measures for developing a culture where the younger members of society look after the older adults, and development of a health insurance and pension schemes will be helpful[78].

Finally, training of medical and paramedical staff to understand the special health needs of the elderly is required. The retraining of healthcare professionals to allay their prejudices concerning old age and those elderly should be implemented in a strategic manner.

The healthcare setup may need to be overhauled to shift its focus from symptomatic treatment and relief to implement the measures to slow down ageing by preventive measures such as immunization against influenza and stress on health promotion measures like nutritional supplementation will go a long way in warding off disease and disability.

CHAPTER SEVENTEEN

THE SUCCESSFUL AGEING:
Staying Alive and Well

AGEING SUCCESSFULLY

Successful ageing has been defined as one's ability to maintain a physically healthy state, mental and physical functioning, and social engagement[79]. The absence of either physical disease or physical disability is not a prerequisite for successful ageing. The people having a physical illness or physical disability can be ageing successfully. Those having diabetes, high blood pressure, arthritis, heart disease, stroke and even cancer can also be ageing successfully. But an optimal functioning of the brain and mind is the primary component of successful ageing. Those suffering from dementia or a severe mental illness cannot be said to be ageing successfully even if otherwise physically healthy.

The successful ageing has certain essential components such as biological health, mental health, cognitive efficiency, social competence, productivity, personal control and physical independence and life satisfaction. Further, these components are mutually interactive and dynamic. Studies show that age-related cognitive decline, even in the absence of dementia or MCI, can impair the activities of daily living (ADL). Thus, to facilitate successful cognitive aging is an essential aspect of successful aging.

There exists a stigma about ageing. There is a common belief that ageing is associated with loss of ability, illness, dementia, and depression. Many think that life goes a downhill course in old age. With this kind of pessimistic attitude towards ageing, people fail to realize that the population is growing older, and there are increasing numbers of people who are leading healthy and functional lives well into older years and coping with ageing successfully.

THE PLASTICITY OF AGEING

Certain things are important such as the healthy behaviours (avoidance of smoking, drinking, violent behavior etc.), physical activities such as exercise, and mental activities like participation in decision making for successful ageing. The resilience is important, and the way people adapt to the changes of ageing varies. Different people react differently to life situations. Certain changes are inevitable with ageing, like loss of mobility due to arthritis, difficulty with vision and hearing, financial stress after retirement, and loss of friends, family members, or even one's spouse. The health-care costs go up, accentuating the stress.

It seems that both genes and environment play a role in ageing successfully. The genes may predispose to diseases and have impact on other things like personality, coping strategies and resilience. But the genes are not everything. Less than 25 percent of longevity is accounted for by genetic factors. The environment and behavior pattern have a significant impact on expression of genes.

Another emerging concept is the neuroplasticity of ageing[80]. The studies show that the brain can continue to grow or develop even in old age. The neuronal regeneration can occur, under certain circumstances, despite ageing. A stimulating environment facilitates regeneration of neurons and favours neuroplasticity of ageing and the successful ageing. The successful ageing, thus, involves a neuro-psychiatric aspect.

CONCEPT OF SUCCESSFUL
AND OPTIMAL AGEING

The research evidence on various aspects of successful ageing suggests ways to maintain optimal physical, mental, and social functioning throughout life by making vital choices that can delay or avoid the diseases and infirmity at advanced age. The lifestyle choices are, as significant as genetic inheritance, for they can determine how well one ages, and have a positive impact on quality of life no matter how late in life they are initiated.

In toto, the concept of successful ageing is, important for assisting people in delaying and preventing various age-related diseases, ageing slowly, and living a healthy and productive life. The elements of optimal ageing are: a high physical functioning, a high mental or cognitive functioning, an active social functioning, and the overall health.

1. High Physical Activity

Physical activity is essential to physical, cognitive, and social functioning as well as to overall health. It is, thus, a primary factor for promoting optimal ageing. The adequate physical activity, even if initiated in later years, contributes to a high physical and cognitive functioning, the overall health, and satisfying engagement with life. It contributes to muscle strength and tone, flexibility, cardiovascular health and positive mood. A regular participation in moderate intensity physical activity is associated with longevity and well-being.

Conversely, the physical inactivity has been associated with muscle atrophy, reduced endurance and muscle strength, and increased mortality. As such, the physical inactivity leads to decrease in physical function and recreational and social opportunities and enhances disability and dependence on others for assistance with activities of daily living.

2. Wholesome Nutrition

A healthy nutrition delays or prevents chronic diseases in later life and leads to additional years of good health, productivity, and high functioning. However, older adults may be at risk for inadequate nutrition because of physiological changes leading to organ functional declines, which affect digestion, metabolism, and absorption of nutrients. Additionally, the older adults' nutritional intake may be compromised because of development of poor eating habits related to chewing or swallowing difficulties as well as diminished interest in food resulting from sensory loss involving taste and smell.

Many older adults are deficient in particular vitamins and minerals, including vitamins B6, B12, D, K, folic acid, and the antioxidant vitamins A, C, E, and beta carotene, as well as the minerals, such as, selenium, calcium, and iron, which are essential for overall health. A long-term cognitive impairment may occur due to malnutrition. Other nutrients such as antioxidants and vitamin C may be protective against cognitive decline. There is strong evidence that folic acid deficiency can increase risk for coronary artery disease and stroke.

Other dietary factors associated with successful ageing, are consumption of significantly less fat and more of complex carbohydrates. Dietary fibre intake is associated with lowering of blood lipids and sugar levels. Eating a healthy diet assists in weight reduction and alters lipid profile favourably. The optimal calcium intake is related to reducing the risk of bone loss and osteoporosis in both men and women and decreasing the incidence of fractures.

The studies have found that dietary caloric restriction, a reduced over-all food intake - a low-calorie diet (1600-2000 Cal per day), may maximize life spans and positively affect ageing and prevent infirmity (Fig 31).

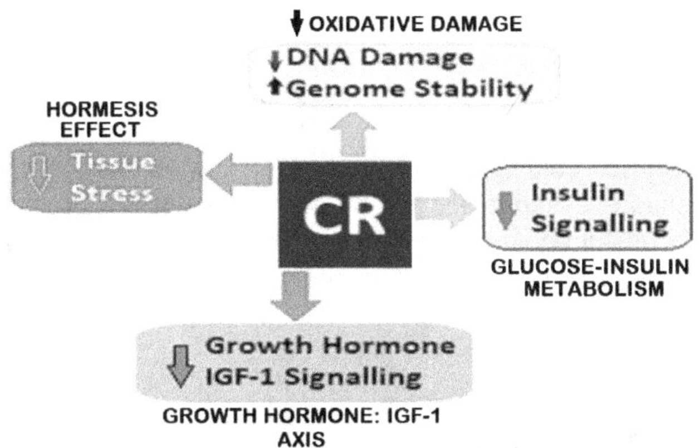

Figure 31: CR Adequate Nutrition and Longevity Circuits

Furthermore, the caloric restriction has been found to decrease the risk of the most age-related diseases, including cardiovascular disease, diabetes, and cancers; delay age-related functional deficits in the brain; reduce the risk of major neuro-degenerative disorders including Alzheimer's disease and Parkinson's disease; and promotes successful ageing.

3. Active Social Support

The social support is an important factor in health promotion and maintenance. It contributes to better physical and cognitive functioning and supporting engagement with life. A good social support leads to healthy behaviours. It also aids in recuperating from an illness. Epidemiological data confirm that social support, that is, good social relationships and a strong social network, is related to longevity and reduced morbidity. Being social promotes better eating and likelihood of continuing physical activity behaviours and assists in warding off alienation and depression.

The older adults who are socially engaged with others and participate in solving daily problems stay in a good cognitive state. Conversely, social dis-engagement in cognitively intact elders is found to be an independent risk factor for cognitive decline. The support of family and friends is essential for an active, emotionally secure, and successful ageing. Moreover, the continued participation in work activity and other events after retirement plays an important role in maintaining cognitive reserve and vitality, and in promoting healthy behaviours.

THE EVALUATION OF LIFE-STYLE PATTERNS

This helps in planning prevention or minimization of risks to health, and in maintenance of a good physical, cognitive, and social functioning by identifying and alleviating the disordered patterns. On the basis of the evaluation, suggestions can be made for positive lifestyle related behavioral changes.

➢ The Physical Activity Scale for the Elderly (PASE) can examine daily activity level and general exercise participation.

➢ The Nutritional Risk Index: Takes into account the dimensions of nutritional risk, namely, mechanics of food intake, prescribed dietary restrictions, conditions affecting food intake, discomfort in food intake, and significant changes in dietary intake.

➢ The Mini-Nutritional Assessment uses anthropometric (e.g., height, weight, etc.), dietetic, and subjective assessments. It identifies the older adults in three categories: those having normal or adequate nutrition, those at risk for malnutrition, and those who are undernourished.

ACTION PLAN
FOR HEALTHY AGEING

The older adults can live longer life in healthier way by working with their family members and health care providers to manage their situations. The first step is planning for minimizing identified health risks. There should be a daily provision of exercise. One should take religiously the prescribed medications and go for regular health check-ups.

When illness is detected, the prescribed treatment should be properly followed. Often, many people fail to follow the entire treatment regimen prescribed by their doctor. For example, nearly one in five older adults with diabetes, skips medication, and has a poorer diabetes control, leading to a worse physical and mental functioning. The studies show that over 75 percent of older adults who fail to take prescribed medications are likely to experience a significant decline in their overall health.

Most of the chronic diseases can be treated or managed well if they are detected in time. A regular follow-up will ensure timely changes in the treatment and life-style advice, ensuring healthy ageing. Encouraging timely health check-ups and screening tests is, thus, vital in this context.

PART SEVEN

<u>ACHIEVING LONGEVITY</u>

CHAPTER EIGHTEEN
GUIDELINES FOR LIFE BEAUTIFUL
Diet & Nutrition. Activity & Exercise.
Medications for Rejuvenation.
Ancillary Measures

195--219

CHAPTER EIGHTEEN

GUIDELINES FOR LIFE BEAUTIFUL: Diet & Nutrition. Activity & Exercise. Medications for Rejuvenation. Ancillary Measures.

THE GENERAL
LIFESTYLE ADVISORY

Ageing is a complex process and affects virtually all organs of the body. Thinking rationally, it is unlikely that something like a pill or potion can reverse the changes and dysfunctions associated with ageing. Thus, rationalizing the outlook is crucial. Any drug or herb advertised and assigned various benefits, in fact, may not help and prove harmful. Losing faith in magic cures is important for rationalizing the approach to protect your health by not becoming yourself a guinea pig for the inadequately researched drugs, phony concoctions, and ill-defined potions. The irrational hopes move you away from terra ferma and are detrimental to rational scientific behavior.

The lifestyle habits play a huge role in keeping the body and mind healthy and fit well into the eighth and ninth decades of life. Of course, researchers cannot guarantee that people who make lifestyle changes will live to the age of 100. But the findings from various studies suggest that most people can live well past 65 and after.

The best way to lead a long and healthy life is to keep fit and prevent and deal effectively with the chronic diseases. In addition, certain simple lifestyle changes are of prime importance. They consist of changes in dietary habits, a regular physical exercise, quitting unhealthy habits like smoking, drinking and violent behavior, and developing a positive attitude. Maintaining close ties with family and friends is helpful. The living arrangement should be such that it fosters physical activity and social relations, and promotes personal health and well-being.

Finally, finding the ongoing meaning to life and fulfilment, or as they call *ikegai* in Japanese, matters to make the life beautiful (Fig 32).

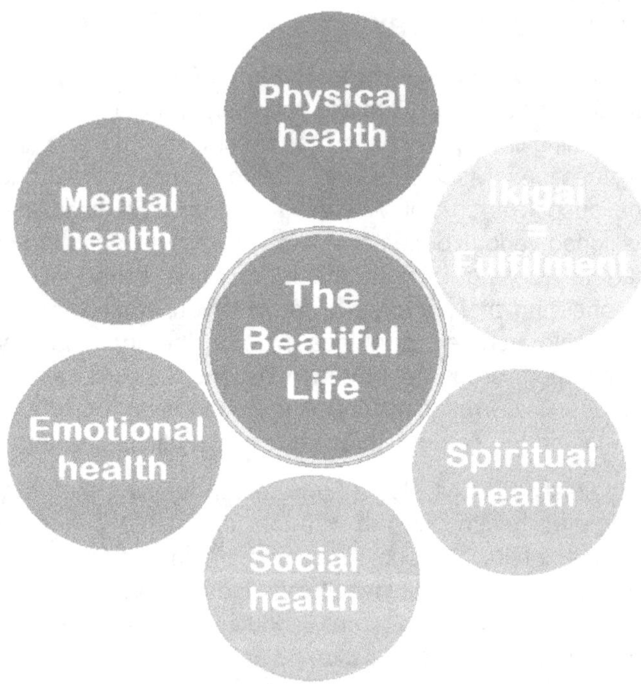

Figure 32: The components of the *Life Beautiful*

WORKING FOR FITNESS AND HEALTH

• <u>Lose weight</u>: An ideal body weight is desirable. Extra weight puts a strain on the heart and other body organs. Overweight and obesity put people at risk of heart attacks, diabetes, cancer and other diseases that can shorten life. The cutting down on calories and trimming the waistline can help in extending life. New research suggests animals that are fed far fewer calories live about 40 percent longer. The same can be applicable to humans.

• <u>Learn something new</u>: Doing something new helps the brain. People, who learn new skills or get new information probably, stimulate the building of new brain cells and connections between existing neurons.

• <u>Exercise and shaping up</u>: The regular exercises help in preventing or delaying many diseases including, heart disease, colon cancer, diabetes and Alzheimer's disease. A routine recommendation is for at least 30 minutes of moderately intense exercise 5 days a week or more.

It is never too late to start. Even the older adults, who have never been active before can work up to a fitness routine that will help keep them strong for years to come. Walking, jogging or simply gardening and housework can help people stay in shape. The research shows that most people lose over 20 percent of their muscle mass by age 70, leading to infirmity. People can reverse this aspect of ageing by regular exercising.

• <u>If you smoke, stop</u>: Smoking is harmful in all age groups. It is more so in the older adults. Many of them already have respiratory problems, diabetes, high blood pressure, and heart disease. Here, smoking can exacerbate the disease.

• <u>Go and Socialize</u>: Going out to meet people, to a party, joining a club, an outing, or a picnic, are some of the many ways to socialize. Those, who build and maintain friendships and family relationships are often healthier and seem to recover faster from illness. Apart from physical and mental health, there are emotional, social and spiritual aspects of health, the superstructures to basic health, which too are to be taken care of (Fig 33).

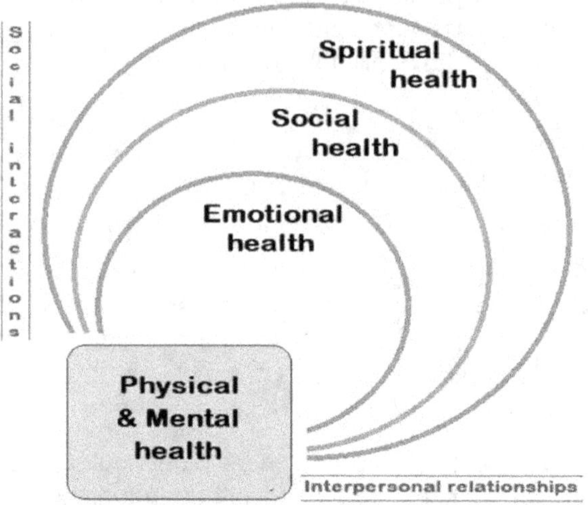

Figure 33: Superstructures to physical and mental health

• <u>Reduce stress</u>: Taking a walk, praying, meditating or having lunch with a friend, are some of the stress-busting measures. People, who build the stress-busting habits into their daily routine, benefit much. Unhealthy stress puts people at risk of getting sick, ageing faster and developing chronic disorders that can cut life short. Social interactions ward off depression and seem to boost the body's immune system.

• <u>Adopt coping mechanisms</u>: The attitude to daily life events is important. The attitudes generate emotional reactions, which affect immune system, circulatory system and even risk of accidents. The attitudes can be improved or changed with training and the beneficial effects be accrued. Research shows that people who live to be 100 often have a happy-go-lucky personality or have well-developed coping mechanisms. An optimistic approach is helpful.

• <u>Eat a healthy diet</u>: Diets that include servings of fruits and vegetables everyday help prevent age-related damage to cells. They contain protective substances that might help in warding off diseases such as cancer and heart disease. Cutting down on fatty and salty foods, and taking whole grain foods, will certainly help.

• <u>Get a good night's sleep</u>: The sleep deprivation can lead to memory lapses, depression and decreased immunity, and hastens neuronal ageing. This can affect health adversely, in general.

• <u>Get a health check-up</u>: A regular health check-up helps in discovering diseases like diabetes, high blood pressure, heart disease and cancers. They can be treated and their complications can be prevented if they are diagnosed in time.

EMBRACING THE RIGHT LIFESTYLE CHOICES

1. <u>Moderate Alcohol Intake</u>: Several studies show that moderate alcohol intake may help to protect against heart disease. But the optimal word is moderate. Excessive alcohol intake can lead to liver damage, drug interactions and injury.

2. <u>No Smoking</u>: Smoking contributes to heart disease, circulatory problems and can cause emphysema and lung cancer. Quitting smoking is fundamental to staying in better health. So, quit if you smoke.

3. <u>Exercise</u>: A 30 minutes of moderate exercise daily for most people is good. The exercise can be as simple as walking, jogging or biking. All exercise programs should

include a weight bearing exercise to help keep bones strong.

4. <u>Appropriate Weight</u>: Overweight and obesity are bad for health. They can contribute to heart disease, diabetes, and joint problems. Moderation in food intake is the most sensible way to maintain weight in the ideal range.

5. <u>Positive Coping Mechanisms</u>: Learning how to control stress and deal with anger can dramatically improve the quality of life. Yoga and Meditation are excellent ways to relax. It is a stressful world, but we can learn to cope. The positive attitudes help. In fact, the prospects for a healthy and long life are dependent upon mental habits.

6. <u>Stable Marriage</u>: A good marriage needs mutual love and commitment. The studies show that happily married people live longer. The marital problem may need counselling. A sexual dysfunction needs to be treated. If the spouse has died, trying to stay socially active in community may help. Friendships can develop and fill in the gaps in one's life.

7. <u>Depressive Illness</u>: A depressive illness deteriorates the quality of life. Your family member, friends, or yourself, may identify if a depressive tendency persists for abnormal period. If you suffer with depression, seek advice, and follow treatment.

**FINDING DOCTORS
WHO CARE**

• As you age, you need to redefine your health needs and priorities. You need to find a doctor, whom you can trust and who understands your health problems and aware of your clinical history. He should be located in the vicinity and available in hours of need.

• You can make a list of what you want in a doctor as a person and as your medical advisor. Consider finding a doctor who listens to you attentively and answers your questions, explaining things clearly. He should speak your language. Often there is a difficulty   in   understanding your   doctor because he uses medical jargons. He should speak a language, which you can understand. This is imperative for following your doctor's instructions as well as understanding about your health problem.

• Type of doctor you need: Deciding the type of doctor you need, is a way to narrow down your choices.

Types of doctors you might consider include: General practitioners- These doctors treat a wide variety of health problems. They do not specialize in one area of medicine. Family practitioners- These doctors provide care for all ages. They are a popular choice if you want a doctor to look after the health of your entire family. Physicians or internists - Internists provide care for adults only, covering a wide spectrum of disorders. Specialists- Specialists are internists with additional training in a particular medical field. For example, a cardiologist is specially trained to treat heart problems.

General practitioners, family practitioners and general internists provide the primary care. They treat diseases and conditions but also advise you on how to prevent health problems. On the other hand, specialists provide care about a specific disease.

• It is worthwhile to check your new doctor's credentials. This can be done in various ways. Check about the doctor's education and training, and his experience with the chronic health conditions you might have. Make sure, who will see you or answer your calls when he is out of town.

Finding a suitable doctor may seem a bit difficult. But it will offer a good level of satisfaction when you turn to him for medical advice in the future. Once you have selected a doctor, make an appointment to talk with him about your medical history. Once you have decided about the suitable doctor, find a local hospital where you can be admitted in future for an illness that requires indoor treatment. Your doctor can help you in this regard.

THE PROTECTIVE EFFECTS OF EXERCISE

Various studies prove that a regular exercise doubtlessly enable to live longer. It is recommended that all older adults should exercise for a minimum of 30 minutes, preferably daily. The exercise should be accomplished in daily increments of as little as five to ten minutes.

The regular exercise is associated with a lower death rate. The lowering of mortality occurs, not only from heart disease, but, from all causes. In a study, there was a 40 percent reduction in heart attacks in females and a 60 percent reduction in heart attacks in males. There is a benefit of exercise for those taking up exercise, even after the age of 60, in form of increase in the life expectancy.

With ageing there is risk of cognitive decline due to the process of neurodegeneration resulting in mild cognitive impairment or more severe diseases such as Parkinson's disease and Alzheimer's disease. The exercise enhances blood flow in brain, neurogenesis, and brain plasticity, it may serve as a potential therapeutic tool to prevent, delay, or treat cognitive decline[81]. In fact, it has been reported that the older adults actually gain more in mental performance from exercise than younger adults. The older women benefit more from increased physical activity as they age than do men. The reason for that appears to be hormonal.

By a regular exercise, apart from heart disease, other diseases like colon cancer are also reduced. The incidence of breast cancer is significantly reduced in females who regularly exercise during the childbearing years. Osteoporosis is reduced by exercise, which increases bone density and improves strength as well as balance, and reduces the risk of falls and fracture. The exercise boosts up the immune system. Another advantage of exercise is its positive impact on the treatment of depression.

Exercise: Key to Activism

• Engaging in regular physical activity and improving sedentary habits promote health and a healthy body weight.

• To reduce the risk of chronic diseases, engage in at least 30 minutes of moderate-intensity physical activity, above usual activity, at work or home on most days of the week[82].

• To prevent weight gain and for sustained weight loss, approximately 60 minutes of moderate to vigorous intensity activity on most days of the week while not exceeding caloric intake requirements, will help[83].

• Achieve physical fitness by including cardiovascular conditioning, stretching exercises for flexibility, and resistance exercises or calisthenics for muscle strength and endurance. Participate in regular physical activity to reduce functional declines associated with ageing.

Exercise and Cardio-Protection

The incidence of angina and myocardial ischemia events, due to the inherent coronary artery disease, is highest in older adults. Regular exercises have been confirmed as a practical countermeasure to protect against the ischemic cardiac injury.

Proposed mechanisms to explain the cardio-protective effect of exercise include the production of myocardial heat-shock protein and other cardio-protective proteins, and improved cardiac antioxidant capacity[84]. These changes lead to an improved heart physiology, resulting in a reduced cardiac ageing. The physical activity has beneficial effects on the heart strength in general.

MEETING ADEQUATE NUTRIENTS AND CALORIE NEEDS

• Consume a variety of nutrient-dense foods and beverages from the basic food groups while choosing foods that limit the intake of saturated and trans fats, cholesterol, added sugars, salt, and alcohol.

• Meet recommended intakes within energy needs by adopting a balanced eating pattern.

• Older adults should consume vitamin B12 in form of supplements[85].

• Older adults with dark skin, and those exposed to insufficient sunlight should consume extra vitamin D from fortified foods or supplements.

THE DIETARY ADVISORY

We need to eat in moderation, and our diet should be varied and internally balanced. This means ingesting the required amounts of calories from each category. The ageing begins much earlier than the middle age and is influenced by genetic factors and actions taken by individuals to address external or exogenous factors including the nutritional requirements[86].

The ageing is also connected with oxidative stress or the generation of free radicals. The free radicals are electrically charged molecules having capacity to chemically react with other molecules. They, also, perform some important cell functions related to metabolism[87]. But, if generated in excess, they can damage certain important biomolecules, such as proteins and other materials associated with the DNA, which deteriorate the cellular reproductive capacity.

To prevent ourselves from the potential damage from excess free radical generation, we should avoid excesses in our lifestyle. Dietary supplementation of antioxidants, including all the vitamins: B, C, A and E and some nutritious minerals such as copper, selenium, manganese, and zinc, can help when required.

A healthy diet should include fruits and vegetables containing nutritious and chemical elements called phyto-chemicals. Over 7000 varieties of phyto-chemicals are known, and they incorporate certain antioxidant agents[88]. A healthy diet containing these elements may help in delaying biological ageing.

THE DIETARY GUIDELINES

There is an emphasis on scientific advice to promote health and reduce risk associated with major chronic diseases through diet and physical activity. A poor diet and a sedentary lifestyle deteriorate health and expose to various disorders. Some specific diseases linked to poor diet and physical inactivity include cardiovascular disease, adult-onset diabetes, hypertension, osteoporosis, and certain cancers. Furthermore, the poor diet and physical inactivity contribute to overweight and obesity which exacerbate complications related to chronic diseases.

The nutrient needs are met through consuming foods. Foods provide nutrients and other compounds that are beneficial for health. In certain cases, fortified foods and dietary supplements may be useful. But, in general, the dietary supplements should not replace a healthful diet.

The recommended calorie intake differs for individuals based on age, gender, and activity level. At each calorie level, individuals who eat nutrient-dense foods may meet their recommended nutrient intake without consuming their full calorie allotment. The remaining calories, the discretionary calorie allowance, allow individuals flexibility to consume some foods and beverages that may contain added fats, added sugars, and alcohol[89].

To maintain body weight in a healthy range, balance calories from foods and beverages with those expended. To achieve gradual weight loss over time, make small decreases in food and beverage calories and increase physical activity.

FOODS TO BE ENCOURAGED

Consume an adequate amount of fruits and vegetables while staying within energy needs. Choose a variety of fruits and vegetables. Selecting from all five vegetable subgroups - dark green, orange, legumes, starchy vegetables, and other vegetables – is simple and helpful. Two servings of fruit and 2-3 bowls of vegetables per day are recommended.

Consume a good number of whole-grain products per day. In general, at least half the grains should come from whole grains. Consume 3 cups per day of fat-free or low-fat milk or equivalent milk products.

SETTING LIMIT ON FOOD COMPONENTS

The total fat intake should be between 20 to 35 percent of calories, with most fats coming from polyunsaturated and monounsaturated fatty acids (fish, nuts and vegetable oils). Less than 10 percent of calories should come from saturated fatty acids. Limit daily cholesterol intake (to less than 300 mg) and trans fatty acid consumption. When selecting meat, poultry, milk and milk products, take care that they are low-fat or fat-free.

Consume less than 2.5 g (approximately 1 tsp of salt) of sodium per day. Choose and prepare foods with low salt content. At the same time, consume potassium-rich foods, such as fruits and vegetables. The older adults and those suffering from high B.P. should not consume more than 1.5 g of sodium per day and meet the potassium recommendation (4,700 mg/day) with food. Choose fibre-rich fruits, vegetables, and whole grains often. Choose and prepare foods and beverages with low sugars.

THE PHYTOCHEMICALS

Phytochemicals are derived from plants and are versatile sources of antioxidants, which enhance the body's defences against harmful reactive oxygen species generated endogenously or exogenously. Tocols, flavonoids, phenolic acids, and ginsenosides are such compounds. The studies have proved that dietary supplementation of phytochemicals has beneficial effects against certain types of pathogens, disease like cancer, and ageing[90]. These effects are related to their ability to boost the antioxidant defence system and reduce oxidative stress. Their excess consumption can have certain adverse effects, too.

ALCOHOLIC BEVERAGES:
RED WINE AND LONGEVITY

Some important biological effects have been attributed to wines in general, but mainly to red wine because of its high content of antioxidants. It has been claimed that red wine could contribute to extending life up to 120 years or more. But its consumption should be in moderation and accompanied by a good quality food.

A scientific investigation carried out in France in 1989, which was sponsored by the World Health Organization, discovered that there are fewer cases of cardiovascular disease in France than in Britain and the United States, because the French regularly consume more red wine and take a diet rich in fruits and vegetables. Reliable scientific literature also attests to the benefits of red wine. The wine is recommended in moderation, along with a balanced diet[91].

The recommendations are:

• If you choose to drink alcoholic beverages, stick to moderation. The limit is consumption of up to one drink per day for women and up to two drinks per day for men.

• Alcoholic beverages should not be consumed if you are taking medications that can interact with alcohol or suffer from specific medical conditions, such as liver disease.

• Avoid alcoholic beverages when engaging in activities that require concentration and attention such as driving.

FOOD SAFETY RECOMMENDATIONS

The food safety is important. The food consumed should be wholesome and free of contamination from infecting agents. To avoid a microbial food-borne illness, clean hands, food contact surfaces frequently, and wash fruits and vegetables. Cook foods to a safe temperature to kill microorganisms. Refrigerate perishable food promptly and defrost foods properly. Do not eat stored food as such.

Do not eat or drink raw milk or any products made from un-pasteurized milk, raw or partially cooked eggs. Avoid foods containing raw or undercooked meat and poultry, raw or undercooked fish or shellfish, unpasteurized juices, and raw sprouts.

THE SIMPLE WAYS FOR STAYING YOUTHFUL

1. Eat a healthy diet, replenished with dietary supplements: Regularly taking vitamin C (1200 mg/day), vitamin E (400 IU/day), calcium (1000-1200 mg/day), vitamin D (400-600 IU/day), folate (400 mcg/day), and vitamin B6 (6 mg/day) can make you look younger and energetic.

2. Quit Smoking and tobacco chewing: Smoking makes you look older by 8 years or more.

3. Control your BP and diabetes: Ideally the control should be to the ideal levels. Controlling to near-ideal levels is a second choice. A person with low blood pressure (~120/80 mm Hg) looks much younger than one with high blood pressure (greater than 140/90 mm Hg).

4. Reduce Stress: By building supporting social networks and adopting stress-busting strategies, you can look younger as well as keep energetic.

5. Taking care of Teeth and oral cavity: Flossing and brushing daily makes you look younger.

6. Be Active: Even a small amount of exercise, for example, 20-minute walk per day helps you look younger, and boosts energy level.

7. Avoid accidents: Regularly wearing a helmet or seat belt and driving within the speed limit relax you and avoid accidents and undesirable consequences.

8. Care of bowels: Taking a moderate amount (25 grams) of fibre in the diet, ensures a good bowel movement and relieves constipation. It helps in lowering cholesterol and precipitous rise in blood sugar level after meals.

9. Monitor Your Health: One should actively seek optimal health care when needed. An optimal treatment slows ageing and improves length as well as quality of life.

10. Laugh a Lot: Laughter reduces stress, strengthens the immune system, and restores youthful energy.

11. Become a Lifelong Learner: People who remain intellectually involved throughout their lives, retard the ageing of their brain.

12. Limit your sex life: Reasonably limiting the sex life not only protects from exposure to venereal infections and dreaded diseases like AIDS; it also helps in keeping emotional balance and conserves energy which can be directed to a creative sphere. A monogamous relationship is the recommended one.

ANCILLARY MEASURES FOR LONGEVITY

Realizing the dream of ageing slowly and living longer involves not only diet, exercise, and curtailing unhygienic habits and choosing healthy habits, it involves help from certain special ways like yoga and T'ai Chi Chuan, also. These ancillary measures help in various ways.

Yoga and Longevity

The yoga is the Hindu philosophical system attributed to Patanjali, who believed in the mystical union of soul with the god through the practice of self-hypnosis and rising above the sense by abstract meditation, adoption of special postures, and ascetic practices. It is a form of spiritual discipline, through which one strives to free the mind from attachment to the senses and achieve a state of calm. The practice of hatha yoga, based on physical postures and control has become increasingly popular.

As practiced in the modern times, yoga is a system of mental and physical exercise, and induced relaxation as a means of relieving stress. Yoga is said to benefit variously. It modifies the secretion of endorphins leading to relief of stress and perhaps modifies various hormones leading to mental fitness and physical including cardiovascular benefits[92].

T'ai Chi Chuan

The Chinese procedure, T'ai Chi Chuan, is considered a soft style martial art and done with as complete a relaxation or softness in the musculature as possible. It is practiced for the purposes of health and longevity. T'ai Chi helps in achieving release of physical and mental stress. It is said to slow ageing and improve physical fitness[93].

The T'ai Chi techniques involve two primary features: the first being the solo form - a slow sequence of movements which emphasize a straight spine, relaxed breathing and a natural range of motion; the second being different styles of pushing hands and sensitivity in the reflexes through various motions which are done in concert with a training partner.

MEDICAL INTERVENTIONS
FOR LONGEVITY

CR WITH NUTRITIONAL SUPPLEMENTATION

So far, it is the only scientifically proved measure to achieve longevity. It calls for restricting the calories consumption - diets having about 30 percent fewer calories, but rich in fruits and vegetables, thus adequate in the nutrients. The hypothesis is based on studies in animals, including rats, mice, fish, flies and worms, which found that the life span of each species could be extended by reducing the number of calories consumed.

Clinical trials in human volunteers have investigated the issue and it appears to apply for human beings also. The studies following underweight people - not those specifically on a calorie-restricted diet - show that they have a higher risk of certain diseases and death. Reducing the number of calories is a good way to lose weight but restricting the diet to the point that it is bereft of essential nutrients is dangerous. The calorie restriction should, thus, be in moderation along with dietary nutritional supplements.

THE ANTI-AGEING DRUGS

All advertisements sound good; they arouse a wishful thinking and hopes. The advertisements of anti-ageing therapies are no exception. There are big claims and sparse evidence.

The ageing process is not yet fully understood. There are multi-billion scientific projects going on to understand ageing and find ways to reverse the effects of ageing. Let us try to find out the therapies currently considered and advocated, and their scientific basis.

Free radical scavengers or antioxidants: The intracellular processes inside the body generate free radicals, which have a damaging effect on intracellular organs and are believed to contribute to ageing and certain diseases. The free radicals are to be dealt with and neutralized. To neutralize them, the body uses antioxidants - certain vitamins, minerals, and enzymes - which are derived from the food.

It is believed that antioxidants by neutralizing the free radicals can prevent or alter the course of chronic diseases such as heart disease and diabetes, and that of ageing. The common antioxidants include vitamin A, vitamin B-6, vitamin B-12, vitamin C, vitamin E, beta carotene, folic acid and selenium. The best way to get the antioxidants is to eat a variety of fruits and vegetables. Using nutritional supplements can also help.

Anti-ageing hormones: Endocrine glands secrete hormones, which stimulate and regulate functions of the vital organs. A proper secretion and balance of various hormones is necessary for health. The levels of certain hormones decline with age. This decline may be responsible for the ageing process. The hormonal therapy to restore the runaway hormones is second only to vitamin supplements in popularity. The aim here is to restore the hormones that decline with age by hormonal supplements to reverse the ageing process.

The most popular hormones involved for replacement therapy are DHEA, human growth hormone, melatonin, testosterone, and estrogen. Though, there is no convincing research evidence to back up the claims for hormonal supplementation. On the other hand, the inadvertent use carries risks for certain adverse effects.

Some of the hormone supplements include:

<u>Growth hormone</u>: The growth hormone is produced by the pituitary gland. It helps growth in childhood and maintains tissues and organs throughout the life. As we age, our body produces less amount of growth hormone. The level of growth hormone begins to drop in the fourth decade.

The growth hormone supplementation is currently approved to treat adults with true growth hormone deficiency, but not the expected decline in growth hormone due to ageing.

It is not known conclusively that supplementation of growth hormone can prevent ageing[94]. The synthetic growth hormone can help healthy older adults, who have naturally low levels of growth hormone to regain some of their youth and vitality. Supplementing the growth hormone through growth hormone injections can increase muscle mass and reduce the amount of body fat in healthy older adults.

The growth hormone supplementation can cause a number of side effects including swelling, arthritis-like symptom, carpal tunnel syndrome, headache, muscle pains, precipitation of diabetes, abnormal growth of bones and internal organs, atherosclerosis, and high blood pressure.

There are claims that a pill form of growth hormone that produces results similar to the injected form of the drug. Calling these pills, human growth hormone releasers, is unsubstantiated by large number of studies. Some web sites sell homeopathic remedies claiming to contain growth hormone. There is no proof to substantiate that either.

De-hydro-epi-androsterone (DHEA)

This hormone is synthesized in the adrenal glands. The body converts DHEA into the sex hormones, estrogen and testosterone. There occurs a decline of androgen levels including DHEA elderly men[95]. It has been suggested, though there is no conclusive evidence, by proponents of DHEA therapy that it can slow ageing, increase muscle strength and bone density, and improve cognition and immunity and protects against chronic diseases.

Testosterone

Declining levels of this male sex hormone have been linked with common complaints associated with ageing, such as decreased energy and sex drive, muscle weakness and osteoporosis[96]. In older men suffering with ADAM and PADAM with low testosterone levels, the clinically proven benefits of testosterone therapy are small and inconsistent. The testosterone therapy has certain well-documented potentially serious adverse effects[97].

Melatonin

This hormone is produced in the brain and regulates sleep. Proponents claim that its supplementation can slow aging, fight cancer, and enhance sexuality. The underlying mechanisms include antioxidant activity, modulation of melatonin receptors MT1 and MT2, stimulation of apoptosis, regulation of pro-survival signaling and tumor metabolism, inhibition on angiogenesis, metastasis, and induction of epigenetic alteration[98]. Melatonin has also been utilized as adjuvant of cancer therapies.

OTHER SUPPLEMENTS

Many drugs, though ill-proven, are advertised as anti-ageing therapies. They include supplements such as coral calcium, ginseng and echinacea. They are not harmless either. Like, ginseng can increase blood pressure especially in those already suffering from high blood pressure. These supplements are often not assayed by drug controllers, so there is no guarantee of product purity or the amount of active ingredient in a given supplement.

The search for effective, nontoxic natural compounds with antioxidative activity has been intensified in recent years. Ganoderma, a mushroom, is claimed to strengthen the immune system and enhance overall health and longevity of life. It is available in various preparations, ranging from toothpaste to massage cream and beverages.

Spirulina is rich in proteins, mineral, and vitamins, is said to have an antioxidant action and boosts immunity and retards ageing. The extract from Morinzhi, Morinda citrifolia, a wild plant, is said to simulate immune system, regulate cell function and help in regeneration of damaged cells.

LONGEVITY BIO-DRUGS OF
DOUBTFUL VALUE

<u>Bristlecone pines</u>

The bristlecone pines belong to family of pine trees that can reach an age far greater than that of any other living thing known - up to nearly 5,000 years. They consist of three closely related species: Rocky Mountains Bristlecone Pine (Pinus aristata) found in Colorado, New Mexico, and Arizona; Great Basin Bristlecone Pine (Pinus longaeva) found in Utah, Nevada and eastern California; and Foxtail Pine (Pinus balfouriana) in California. Currently, the oldest of them is the Pinus longaeva tree nick-named "Methuselah" and is located in the White Mountains of eastern California.

Bristlecone pines grow very slowly. Its wood is very dense and resinous, and thus resistant to invasion by insects, fungi, and other potential pests. Their extract may help in repairing age-related tissue damage and preventing cancers.

<u>Resveratrol</u>

Resveratrol is a polyphenolic phytoalexin compound. It is found in the skins of certain red grapes, in peanuts, blueberries, some pines and the roots and stalks of Japanese knotweed and giant knotweed. It is now registered as an investigational drug. It is also available as a nutritional supplement. Its amount in food substances varies greatly. Red wine contains approximately 5 mg/L. It exists in two structural isomeric forms: cis- and trans-. Trans-resveratrol can undergo isomerisation to the cis form (the ineffective form) when heated or exposed to UV irradiation. Resveratrol is a solid at room temperature and soluble in ethanol, but only sparingly soluble in water.

Resveratrol has antioxidant properties. It lowers incidence of coronary heart disease and interferes with carcinogenesis. It also possesses anti-angiogenic properties. Resveratrol has been reported to be effective against neuronal cell dysfunction and cell death. Resveratrol significantly extends the lifespan of yeast. Only the trans-form of resveratrol is capable of activating the mammalian SIRT1 gene in vitro[99]. Resveratrol has also been seen to increase the potency of some antiretroviral drugs in vitro. It also inhibits the development of cardiac fibrosis.

REGENERATIVE MEDICINE

<u>Cloning for Longevity</u>

Apart from caloric restriction, the regenerative medicine is the next concrete step for achieving longevity. The most promising in regenerative medicine is the therapeutic cloning[100]. A new organ can be grown for transplantation using one's own cells. The process would involve transferring the nucleus from a cell to an enucleated human egg, which would then grow in a petri dish to the blastocyst stage. Stem cells would be harvested from the blastocyst and transformed into the desired tissues for transplant.

The regenerative medicine does not stop or slow ageing but corrects the organ dysfunctions and failure and diseases that accompany ageing. It is just an advanced form of conventional medicine.

<u>Dealing with Free Radicals</u>

The true solution of ageing lies in stopping the free radicals from damaging DNA and cross-linking the important biological molecules. The most popular anti-ageing regimen, practiced by millions, is taking the antioxidant vitamin and mineral pills. There is no firm scientific evidence that such supplements actually increase the life span.

<u>Dealing with Intracellular Gunk</u>

Another way is to break apart advanced glycation end-products, is enabling the cells to get rid of them[101]. A compound called pimagedine has improved cardiac function in rats, dogs, and primates. It is also being tested for efficacy in treating kidney failure associated with diabetes. Another anti-ageing compound, ATL-711, has shown some promise as a treatment to reverse age-related and diabetes-related cardiovascular diseases and restore function to the cardiovascular system.

<u>Restoring Telomerase</u>

Some researchers suggest that it might be possible to stop senescence at the cellular level by getting the cells to produce telomerase, which can prevent the shortening of the telomeres[102]. It will protect them from ageing and rejuvenate them and the tissues in which they reside. The age-related changes of cardiac, endothelial and vascular smooth muscle cells contribute to cardiovascular disease and telomerase therapy may rejuvenate the vascular system[103].

Restoring telomerase can also suitably modify apoptosis or the programmed cell death. There is growing evidence demonstrating the role of apoptosis in chronic diseases like autoimmune disorders, diabetes, Alzheimer's disease and cardiovascular and brain ageing.

THE JEWISH TOAST:
'MAY YOU LIVE TO BE 120'

The possibility of a lengthy-healthy life is alluring. As the life expectancy at birth rises and there is taking place an improvement in average and maximum lifespan, the possibility of living life more than never before seems logical.

The science gives visions; the technology makes the visions possible. The maximum human lifespan was recorded in case of Jeanne Calment, a Frenchwoman, who lived to 122 years. The Jewish toast proclaiming, 'may you live to be 120' is much near the maximum recorded lifespan. It is common among Jews to wish another to live until 120, because as recorded in the Torah 'Moses was 120 years old when he died' (Deuteronomy 34:7).

In light of the progress in health sciences, genetics and biotechnology, it seems very much plausible that a significant extension of lifespan is not a remote dream, but a reasonable possibility in the very-near future.

APPENDICES

Figures in the Book

221-226

Glossary and Abbreviations

227-235

References

236-245

FIGURES IN THE BOOK

Figure 1: Lifestyle choices for healthy longevity

INTRODUCTION
- New, Created for this book.

Figure 2: Age-related decline in functional threshold, performance and productivity.
CHAPTER 3
Nikhra V. COVID-19 Infection in Elderly, Adverse Outcomes and Annihilation of the Longevity Dream. Ann Immunol & Immunoth, 2020, 2(1): 000116. DOI: 10.23880/AII-16000116

Figure 3: IGF and insulin signalling pathway and DAF-2 and DAF-16 transcription factors in C. elegans influencing ageing
CHAPTER
4
Nikhra V. Taming the Pro-Aging Factors and Pathways for Longevity and Improving Health-span. EC Nutrition 15.4 (2020):21-36.

Figure 4. Oxidative stress, DNA damage and ageing link
CHAPTER 4
Nikhra V. COVID-19 Infection in Elderly, Adverse Outcomes and Annihilation of the Longevity Dream. Ann Immunol & Immunoth ISSN: 2691-5782, 2020, 2(1): 000116. DOI: 10.23880/AII-16000116

FIGURE 5: Ageing and testosterone level in men   CHAPTER 6

Nikhra V. The Altered Hormonal Homeostasis with Aging, Neuronal Dysfunction and Cognitive Decline. OAJ Gerontology & Geriatric Medicine 2018; 3(4): 555619. DOI: 10.19080/OAJGGM.2018.03.555619

Figure 6: Cortisol secretion in ageing adults   CHAPTER 7

Nikhra V. The Altered Hormonal Homeostasis with Aging, Neuronal Dysfunction and Cognitive Decline. OAJ Gerontol & Geriatric Med. 2018; 3(4): 555619. DOI: 10.19080/OAJGGM.2018.03.555619

Figure 7: Clinical manifestations of menopause and andropause

CHAPTER 7

Nikhra V. Aging-Related Gonadal Hormonal Deficiency and (Sex)-Hormone Replacement Therapy". EC Endocrinology and Metabolic Research 4.5 (2019): 203-206.

Figure 8. The factors influencing ageing of brain   CHAPTER 8

Vinod N. Aging Brain: Recent Research and Concepts. Gerontol & Geriatric stud. 1(3). GGS.000511. 2017. DOI: 10.31031/GGS.2017.01.000511

Figure 9. The physiological ageing and cognitive decline

CHAPTER 8

Vinod N. Aging Brain: Recent Research and Concepts. Gerontol & Geriatric stud. 1(3). GGS.000511. 2017. DOI: 10.31031/GGS.2017.01.000511

Figure 10: Hypothalamus, neocortex, GNRH and estrogen feedback loop influencing cognitive function.   CHAPTER 8

Vinod Nikhra. The Altered Hormonal Homeostasis with Aging, Neuronal Dysfunction and Cognitive Decline. OAJ Gerontol & Geriatric Med. 2018; 3(4): 555619. DOI: 10.19080/OAJGGM.2018.03.555619

Figure 11: Theories and concepts of neurodegeneration

CAPTER 8

Vinod N. Aging Brain: Recent Research and Concepts. Gerontol & Geriatric stud. 1(3). GGS.000511. 2017. DOI: 10.31031/GGS.2017.01.000511

recruits protein kinase B. PKB signals inhibit FOXO to negatively regulate expression of pro-aging genes and to positively express anti-aging genes. The Sir2 increases longevity by influencing FOXO.

CHAPTER 11

Vinod Nikhra. "Taming the Pro-Aging Factors and Pathways for Longevity and Improving Health-span". EC Nutrition 15.4 (2020): 21-36.

Figure 19: Protective role of STACs in cellular physiology

CHAPTER 11

Vinod Nikhra. "Taming the Pro-Aging Factors and Pathways for Longevity and Improving Health-span". EC Nutrition 15.4 (2020): 21-36.

Figure 20: Adiposity, Stress Factors, p53 and genesis of Metabolic Disorders CHAPTER 11

Vinod N. Metabolic Disequilibrium and Aging: Modifying Favorably with Calorie Restriction and Calorie Restriction Mimetics. Gerontol & Geriatric stud.4(5). GGS.000596.2019. DOI: 10.31031/GGS.2019.04.000596

Fig 21: The stress factors activate p53 by dissociating the mdm2-p53 complex, which influences cell cycle, metabolism, DNA repair, senescence, apoptosis and autophagy and aging process

CHAPTER 11

Vinod N. Metabolic Disequilibrium and Aging: Modifying Favorably with Calorie Restriction and Calorie Restriction Mimetics. Gerontol & Geriatric stud.4(5). GGS.000596.2019. DOI: 10.31031/GGS.2019.04.000596

Figure 22: Metabolic Changes triggered by adiposity.

CHAPTER 11

Vinod Nikhra. The Blueprint for Retarding and Reversing Cardiovascular Aging. OAJ Gerontol & Geriatric Med. 2018; 4(4): 555644. DOI: 10.19080/OAJGGM.2018.04.555644

Vinod Nikhra. The Blueprint for Retarding and Reversing Cardiovascular Aging. OAJ Gerontol & Geriatric Med. 2018; 4(4): 555644. DOI: 10.19080/OAJGGM.2018.04.555644

Figure 29: The social health and spiritual health are often neglected areas in older adults

CHAPTER 16

Modified for the book from - Nikhra V. The Trans-zoonotic Virome interface: Measures to balance, control and treat epidemics. Ann Biomed Sci Eng. 2020; 4: 020-027 DOI: 10.29328/journal.abse.1001009

Figure 30: The effects of Ageing and Disease   CHAPTER 16

From Previous edition of the book – 'Ageing slowly, Living longer'

Figure 31: CR Adequate Nutrition and Longevity Circuits

CHAPTER 17

Vinod N. Future Projections and Fallouts of Exponential Longevity and Revival from Cryopreservation. Res Med Eng Sci. 6(4).   RMES.000640.2018.   DOI: 10.31031/RMES.2018.06.000640

Figure 32: The components of the *Life Beautiful*

CHAPTER 18

- New, Created for this book.

Figure 33: Superstructures to physical and mental health

CHAPTER 18

- New, Created for this book.

GLOSSARY AND ABBREVIATIONS

Adrenopause: State of decline in secretion of adrenal corticoid hormones which include mainly DHEA and DHEA sulphate.

Adrenoreceptors: Receptors for the adrenaline and noradrenaline, the stress hormones.

AGE: Advanced glycation end products, produced by cross linking of large molecules like bioproteins by sugars like glucose.

Alzheimer's disease: Gradual onset dementia of an unknown etiology.

Andropause: State of decline in secretion of testosterone and allied hormones. Similar to menopause in women.

Antigens and antibodies: The immune system recognizes something self and non-self. An antigen is non-self, against which antibodies are produced.

Antioxidants: Compounds that can neutralize reactive oxygen species, ROS, or free radicals.

Apoptosis: A biologically programmed cell death.

Artificial intelligence: Inanimate intelligence as opposed to that possessed by living organisms. Refers to that possessed by computers.

Atherosclerosis: The process of narrowing of arteries by deposition of cholesterol like products inside the arteries.

Auditory canals: Sensitive organs of internal ears.

Baroreceptors: Receptors for regulating pressure of moving blood column.

BMI: A measure involving body weight and height. Used for calculating overweight and obesity.

Botulinum toxin: The lethal toxin produced by bacteria, Clostridium botulinum.

Bristlecone pines: The bristlecone pines belong to family of pine trees that can reach an age far greater than that of any other living thing known - up to nearly 5,000 years. Currently, the oldest of them is the Pinus longaeva tree nick-named "Methuselah".

Cataract: Opacification of eye lens with age.

Chemoreceptors: Sense carbon di oxide and related things in moving blood column.

Chromosomes: The 'threads of life', composed of genes. Lie inside the cell nucleus.

Cloning, therapeutic: Cloning designed as therapy for a disease.

CNS astroglia: The connective tissue of brain.

Cognitive disorders: Defects of brain's higher functions.

Collagen, collagenase, procollagen: Collagen is the connective tissue, procollagen is its precursor, and collagenase is the enzyme.

Coronary heart disease: vastly known as the heart disease. It is essentially due to disturbed blood supply to the heart.

CPR: Cardio-pulmonary resuscitation. To revive the dying patient.

CRAN: The caloric restriction with adequate nutrition.

Cytotoxic factors: Products of inflammation, include IL-1, IL-2, TNF, etc.

DHEA: dehydroepiandrosterone, a hormone

DNA: Building block of genes, which in turn form chromosomes.

Down regulation: Reduced efficacy of a process or receptor.

ED: Erectile dysfunction, a variant of impotence.

Endorphins: Local hormones in brain.

Estrogen, LH, FSH: The female hormones.

FIRKO mouse: Fat insulin receptors knocked out mouse.

Free radicals, ROS: Charge-bearing small molecules, which are highly reactive.

Ganoderma: A mushroom, is claimed to strengthen the immune system and enhance overall health and longevity of life.

Gerontology: The science of study of old age.

Gerontological: Pertaining to old age.

GH: Growth hormone.

Glaucoma: A painful condition of eye due to increased intra-ocular pressure.

Hemoglobin: The red pigment of blood, responsible for carrying oxygen.

Holistic health, the concept of: An all-encompassing health, total health

Hypersensitivity reaction: A severe and sudden allergic reaction.

Immune system: The body's protective system.

Immunosenescence: Deterioration in immunity due to ageing.

Incontinence: Inability to hold or poor control, e.g. that of urine.

Inflammatory process: The reaction following an injury or damage to body tissue.

Inheritance, inheritability: Transfer of biological characteristics from parents to offspring.

Insulin signaling pathway: A metabolic pathway, which could be important in controlling ageing.

Ion channels: Cellular organs controlling entry or exit of charged micro-molecules called ions.

Ischemia: Impending tissue damage due to disruption of blood supply.

Jeanne Calment, a Frenchwoman, who lived to 122 years.

Leptin: Hormone produced by fat cells.

Life beautiful: A concept proposed by the author encompassing holistic health plus meaning to life and fulfilment

Lost horizon: A novel by James Hilton. Published in 1933, was a huge success. The hero, Hugh Conway roams around to find a fictional town, Shangri-La, whose inhabitants enjoy longevity. The book inspired names of many places and two films: directed by Frank Capra (1937) and Charles Jarrott (1973).

Macular degeneration: Degeneration involving the central part of retina.

'May you live to be 120': A Jewish blessing. It is much near the maximum recorded lifespan. It is common among Jews to wish another to live until 120, because as recorded in the Torah 'Moses was 120 years old when he died' (Deuteronomy 34:7).

Melanin: Pigment in skin cells, responsible for dark color.

Melatonin: A hormone produced by posterior pituitary. Supposed to play a significant role in ageing process.

Menopause, perimenopausal, postmenopausal: Menopause is the period of cessation of menses in women. Postmenopausal is the period after that. Perimenopausal is the brief period on either side of the menopause.

Methuselah: Methuselah, also spelled Methushael, Hebrew Bible (Old Testament) patriarch whose life span as recorded in Genesis (5:27) was 969 years; he has survived in legend and tradition as the longest-lived human. Great Basin bristlecone pine (Pinus longaeva) tree, the long-surviving tree has been named after Methuselah in bible, in the White Mountains of Inyo County in eastern California.

Mitochondria: The cell organelle involved in cellular respiration and energy generation. They also produce ROS, implicated in ageing.

Mutation: Mutation means change at the genetic level. They may confer survival advantage or can have a deleterious effect.

Myocardium: The main tissue of heart.

Nanobiotechnology: Biotechnology at molecular level. It holds immense promise of being able to reverse ageing in some remote future.

Nanotechnology: Technology at molecular level.

Neurone, neuronal: Neurones are the nerve cells. Neuronal means pertaining to the heart.

Omega 3 fatty acids: They are cardioprotective as well as have been shown to prevent the diabetic complications also.

Orbicularis oculi, orbicularis oris: The round muscles around eye and mouth respectively.

Osteopenia: Weakness of bones.

Pacemaker cells: The heart has impulse generating cells, called the pacemaker.

Parkinson's disease: The disease also called, shaking palsy, a disorder due to neuronal degeneration.

Plasticity of ageing: describes capacity for change, i.e., an individual's capability and reserve capacity to react to demands of the environment by means of cognitive, behavioral, or any other kind of reorganization. Plasticity may appear at various levels (e.g., brain structure, behavior) and can be related to different domains (e.g., cognitive plasticity, behavioral plasticity, personality plasticity).

Performance anxiety: An apprehension elated to poor sexual prowess. A common accompaniment of ED.

Prostate: The ancillary sexual gland in men. Enlargement of prostate is common in older adult males.

Rejuvenative medicine: The branch of medicine dealing with restoration of youth.

Resveratrol: Resveratrol is a polyphenolic phytoalexin compound. It is found in the skins of certain red grapes, in peanuts, blueberries, etc. It is now an investigational drug.

Regenerative medicine: a branch of translational research in tissue engineering and molecular biology which deals with the "process of replacing, engineering or regenerating human or animal cells, tissues or organs to restore or establish normal function

Roundworms: Belong to worm family, Nematoda. Round worms are often parasites, like Ascaris lumbricoides. Caenorhabditis elegans is a tiny microscopic round worm, found in soil.

Sarcopenia: Weakness of muscles.

Senile brain disease: Senile Degeneration of Brain, also known as senile brain degeneration, is related to posterior cortical atrophy. An important gene associated with Senile Degeneration of Brain is APP (Amyloid Beta Precursor Protein).

SNAPs: Single nucleotide polymorphisms. Very common genetic variations. Often not significant.

Somatopause: Phenomenon due to fall in somatic hormone, commonly known as growth hormone.

Spirulina: Spirulina is a type of blue-green algae that is popular as a supplement. Spirulina is incredibly nutritious, and has numerous health benefits.

Suprachiasmic nuclei: Lie in brain. Important in hormonal regulation.

Suppressor cells: Part of immune system. Apart from memory cells, natural killer cells and activated killer cells.

Synapses: Junctions formed by neurons. Important in neuronal messaging. Work through neurotransmitters.

T'ai Chi Chuan: Tai chi, is a self defense and calisthenics technique developed in China centuries ago as a maturation of several similar but separate exercises. The more formal name of this technique is tai chi chuan, which translates loosely to "supreme ultimate boxing."

Telomere and telomerase: Telomere is the end-genes on a chromosome. Some part is usually lost with every cell division. Where there occurs a significant loss, further cell division is stopped. This controls the limit of cell division. The number is known as Hayflick number. Telomerase, an enzyme, is capable of restoring telomeres.

Thymidine dimmers: Produced during exposure of skin to sunlight. Play an important part in ageing of skin.

Thymus, thymic hormones: Thymus is the hormonal gland, which atrophies early at the beginning of middle age. Thymic hormones play important part in immunity.

Tissues and cells: Cells are the body's building blocks. A specialized group of cells is called tissue.

Tithonus option: Long life with poor quality. A nightmare of trans-humanists. The supposed dark side of life extension.

Type 2 diabetes, adult onset diabetes: The common form of diabetes in adults and older adults.

Unlimited potential: All of us carry unlimited potential, most of which we fail to utilize. Albert Einstein stated that most of us use 5 percent of our brain intelligence. One using about 7 percent can be called an intelligent person.

Visceral obesity: Abdominal obesity.

'Yayati Syndrome': An original connotation for this specific description used by the author.in the 2006 edition of this book.

Many words and terms have been explained in the text as they appear. They have been, hence, not included in the glossary.

REFERENCES

1. 'What A Wonderful World' – A famous lyric, sung by Louis Armstrong and written by George David Weiss, Robert Thiele. (What A Wonderful World/ I see trees of green, red roses too/ I see them bloom for me and you/ And I think to myself what a wonderful world/ I see skies of blue and clouds of white/ The bright blessed day, the dark sacred night/ And I think to myself what a wonderful world/ The colours of the rainbow so pretty in the sky/ Are also on the faces of people going by/ I see friends shaking hands saying how do you do/ .. what a wonderful world).

2. Gavrilov LA, Gavrilova NS. 2004. Early-life programming of aging and longevity: the idea of high initial damage load (the HIDL hypothesis). Ann N Y Acad Sci. 2004,1019:496-501. DOI: 10.1196/annals.1297.091.

3. Klein BJ. 2003. This Wonderful Lengthening of Lifespan. https://www.fightaging.org/archives/2003/01/this-wonderful-lengthening-of-lifespan/

4. In 1962, in his book "Profiles of the Future: An Inquiry into the Limits of the Possible", science fiction writer Arthur C. Clarke formulated his famous Three Laws, of which the third law is the best-known and most widely cited: "Any sufficiently advanced technology is indistinguishable from magic".

5. Vinod N. Future Projections and Fallouts of Exponential Longevity and Revival from Cryopreservation. Res Med Eng Sci. 6(4). RMES.000640.2018. DOI: 10.31031/RMES.2018.06.000640

6. Christensen K, Johnson TE, Vaupel JW. The quest for genetic determinants of human longevity: challenges and insights. Nat Rev Genet. 2006, 7:6; 436–48. DOI: 10.1038/nrg1871.

7. Gabriele D, Jim O. Reproduction and longevity among the British peerage: the effect of frailty and health selection. Proc. R. Soc. Lond. 2003. B.270; 1541-47. DOI: 10.1098/rspb.2003.2400.

8. O'Donnell AB, Araujo AB, McKinlay JB. The health of normally aging men: The Massachusetts Male Aging Study (1987-2004). Exp Gerontol. 2004, 39:7; 975-84. DOI: 10.1016/j.exger.2004.03.023.

9. Dobrzyńska MM, Pachocki KA, Owczarska K. DNA strand breaks in peripheral blood leucocytes of Polish blood donors. 2018. *Mutagenesis*, 33:1, 69–76, DOI: 10.1093/mutage/gex024.

10. Nathan BP, Jiang Y, Wong GK, et al. Apolipoprotein E4 inhibits, and apolipoprotein E3 promotes neurite outgrowth in cultured adult mouse cortical neurons through the low-density lipoprotein receptor-related protein. Brain Res, 2002. 928:1-2; 96-105. DOI 10.1016/s0006-8993(01)03367-4.

11. Morselli E, Santos RS, Criollo A, et al. The effects of oestrogens and their receptors on cardiometabolic health. *Nat Rev Endocrinol.* 2017, 13:6; 352-64. DOI:10.1038/nrendo.2017.12

12. Matsumoto AM. Andropause: Clinical Implications of the Decline in Serum Testosterone Levels with Aging in Men. *The Journals of Gerontology: Series A*, 2002, 57:2, M76–M99, DOI: 10.1093/gerona/57.2.M76

13. El Khoudary SR, McClure CK, VoPham T, et al. Longitudinal assessment of the menopausal transition, endogenous sex hormones, and perception of physical functioning: The Study of Women's Health Across the Nation. Journals of Gerontology, Series A: Biological Sciences and Medical Sciences 69.8 (2014): 1011-17.

14. Marjoribanks J, Farquhar C, Roberts H, et al. Long-term hormone therapy for perimenopausal and postmenopausal women. *Cochrane Database Syst Rev.* 2012, 7:CD004143. DOI: 10.1002/14651858.CD004143.pub4

15. El-Sakka AI, Hassoba HM. Age related testosterone depletion in patients with erectile dysfunction. Journal of Urology, 2006, 176; 2589-93.

16. Panay N, Haitham H, Arya R, et al. British Menopause Society and Women's Health Concern: The 2013 British Menopause Society and Women's Health Concern recommendations on hormone replacement therapy. Menopause International, 2013, 19.2; 59-68.

17. Snyder PJ, Bhasin S, Cunningham GR, et al. Effects of testosterone treatment in older men. New England Journal of Medicine, 2016, 374.7; 611-24, DOI: 10.1056/NEJMoa1506119.

18. Anawalt BD, Yeap BB. Conclusions about testosterone therapy and cardiovascular risk. Asian Journal of Andrology, 2018, 20.2,152-53.

19. Gagliano-Jucá T, Basaria S. Testosterone replacement therapy and cardiovascular risk. Nature Reviews Cardiology, 2019, 16:9; 555-74. DOI: 10.1038/s41569-019-0211-4.
20. Denburg NL, Cole CA, Hernandez M, Yamada TH, Tranel D, et al. (2007) The orbitofrontal cortex, real-world decision-making, and normal aging. Ann N Y Acad Sci, 2007, 1121: 480-98.
21. Tucker AM, Stern Y. Cognitive reserve in aging. Curr Alzheimer Res, 2011, 8:4; 354-360.
22. Scahill R, Frost C, Jenkins R, et al. A longitudinal study of brain volume changes in normal ageing using serial registered magnetic resonance imaging. Arch Neurol, 2003, 60:7; 989-94.
23. Herlitz A, Yonker J. Hormonal effects on cognition in adults. In: New frontiers in cognitive ageing. 2004, Dixon R, Bäckman L, Nilsson L (Eds.), Oxford University Press, India, 253-78.
24. Fratiglioni L, Launer L, Anderson K, et al. Incidence of dementia and major subtypes in Europe: a collaborative study of population-based cohorts. Neurologic Diseases in the Elderly Research Group. Neurology, 2000, 54(11Suppl 5): S10-S15.
25. Lobo A, Launer L, Fratiglioni L, et al. For the Neurologic Diseases in the Elderly Research Group. Prevalence of dementia and major subtypes in Europe: a collaborative study of population based-cohorts. Neurology, 2000, 54(11Suppl 5): S4-S9.
26. Johnson LA, Hobson V, Jenkins M, et al. The Influence of Thyroid Function on Cognition in a Sample of Ethnically Diverse, Rural-Dwelling Women: A Project FRONTIER Study. 2011, 23:2, 219-22.
27. Incidence of CVD by age and sex, Incidence and prevalence 2006; Incidence and Prevalence: 2006 Chart Book on Cardiovascular and Lung Diseases - Nat. Heat, Lung and Blood Inst. Accessed on 19 Feb 2017 at http://www.nhlbi.nih.gov/sites/www.nhlbi.nih.gov/files/06a_ip_chtbk.pdf
28. Roger VL. Go AS, Lloyd-Jones DM, et al. Executive Summary: Heart Disease and Stroke Statistics - 2011 Update: A Report from the American Heart Association. Circulation. 2011; 123: 459–463.

29. North BJ, Sinclair DA. The Intersection between Aging and Cardiovascular Disease; Circ Res. 2012 April 13; 110(8): 1097–1108.
30. Mahmood SS, Levy D, Vasan RS, et al. The Framingham Heart Study and the Epidemiology of Cardiovascular Diseases: A Historical Perspective; Lancet. 2014 Mar 15; 383(9921): 999–1008; Published online 2013.
31. Strait JB, Lakatta EG: Aging-associated cardiovascular changes and their relationship to heart failure; Heart Fail Clin. 2012 Jan; 8(1): 143–164.
32. Benigni A, Corna D, Zoja C, et al. Disruption of the Ang II type 1 receptor promotes longevity in mice. J Clin Invest. 2009, 119: 524–530.

33. Inserra F, Romano L, Ercole L, et al. Cardiovascular changes by long-term inhibition of the renin-angiotensin system in aging. Hypertension 1995, 25: 437–442.

34. Bristow MR. Treatment of Chronic Heart Failure With β-Adrenergic Receptor Antagonists. Circulation Research. 2011, 109; 1176–94, DOI: 10.1161/CIRCRESAHA.111.245092
35. Moslehi J, DePinho RA, Sahin E. Telomeres and Mitochondria in the Aging Heart Circ. Res. 2012, 110; 1226-37.
36. La'hteenvuo J, Rosenzweig A. Effects of Aging on Angiogenesis, Circulation Research 2012, 110; 1252-64.
37. Halaschek-Wiener J, Khattra JS, McKay S, et al. Analysis of long-lived C. elegans daf-2 mutants using serial analysis of gene expression. *Genome Res.* 2005, 15:5; 603-15. DOI: 10.1101/gr.3274805
38. Park CB, Larsson NG. Mitochondrial DNA mutations in disease and aging. J Cell Biol 2011, 193:5; 809-18. DOI: 10.1083/jcb.201010024.
39. Doblhammer G, Vaupel JW. Lifespan depends on month of birth. Proc Natl Acad Sci U S A. 2001, 98:5; 2934-39. DOI: 10.1073/pnas.041431898
40. Gavrilov L.A., Gavrilova N.S. Human Longevity and Parental Age at Conception. In: Sex and Longevity: Sexuality, Gender, Reproduction, Parenthood. Research and Perspectives in Longevity. 2001. Eds - Robine JM, Kirkwood TBL and Allard

M. 2001. Springer, Berlin. DOI: 10.1007/978-3-642-59558-5_2

41. Vågerö D, Aronsson V, Modin B. Why is parental lifespan linked to children's chances of reaching a high age? A transgenerational hypothesis. SSM Popul Health. 2017, 4; 45-54. DOI: 10.1016/j.ssmph.2017.11.006

42. Kenyon C. The first long-lived mutants: discovery of the insulin/IGF-1 pathway for ageing. Philos Trans R Soc Lond B Biol Sci. 2011, 366: 1561, 9–16, DOI: 10.1098/rstb.2010.0276

43. Weindruch R, Sohal RS. Caloric Intake and Aging. N Engl J Med. 1997 337:14; 986–994. DOI: 10.1056/NEJM199710023371407

44. Dato S, Soerensen M, De Rango F, et al. The genetic component of human longevity: New insights from the analysis of pathway-based SNP-SNP interactions. Aging Cell. 2018, 17:3; e12755. DOI: 10.1111/acel.12755

45. Gavrilov L, Gavrilova N. The Reliability Theory of Aging and Longevity. Journal of Theoretical Biology, 2001, 213:4; 527-545. DOI: 10.1006/jtbi.2001.2430

46. Mitteldorf J. What Is Antagonistic Pleiotropy? Biochemistry Moscow 2019, 84; 1458–68. DOI: 10.1134/S0006297919120058

47. van den Heuvel J, English S, Uller T. Disposable Soma Theory and the Evolution of Maternal Effects on Ageing. PLoS One. 2016, 11:1; e0145544. DOI: 10.1371/journal.pone.0145544

48. Goldsmith TC. Aging as an Evolved Characteristic - Weismann's Theory Reconsidered. Medical Hypotheses Version, 2003, 62:2, 304-308 2004. DOI: 10.1016/S0306-9877(03) 00337-2

49. Lee AC, Fenster BE, Ito H, et al. Ras proteins induce senescence by altering the intracellular levels of reactive oxygen species. J. Biol. Chem. 1999, 274; 7936-40.

50. Holzenberger M. Igf-I signaling and effects on longevity. Nestle Nutr Workshop Ser Pediatr Program. 2011, 68; 237-45. doi: 10.1159/000325914.

51. Pan H, Finkel T. Key proteins and pathways that regulate lifespan. J Biol Chem. 2017, 292:16; 6452–60. DOI: 10.1074/jbc.R116.771915.

52. Wątroba M, Szukiewicz D. The role of sirtuins in aging and age-related diseases. Adv. Med. Sci. 2016, 61; 52–62.

53. Mitchell SJ, Martin-Montalvo A, Mercken EM, et al. Calorie restriction-like effects of 30 days of resveratrol supplementation on energy metabolism and metabolic profile in obese humans. Cell Metab. 2014, 14, 612–22.
54. Albert V, Hall MN. mTOR signaling in cellular and organismal energetics. Curr. Opin. Cell Biol. 2015, 33; 55–66.
55. Saxton RA, Sabatini DM. mTOR Signaling in Growth, Metabolism, and Disease. Cell. 2017, 168:6; 960-76. DOI: 10.1016/j.cell.2017.02.004
56. Krstic J, Reinisch I, Schupp M, et al. p53 Functions in Adipose Tissue Metabolism and Homeostasis. Int J Mol Sci. 2018, 19:9; 2622. DOI:10.3390/ijms19092622
57. Minamino T, Orimo M, Shimizu I, et al. A crucial role for adipose tissue p53 in the regulation of insulin resistance. Nat Med. 2009, 15:9; 1082-87. DOI:10.1038/nm.2014
58. Hunter GR, Singh H, Carter SJ, et al. Sarcopenia and Its Implications for Metabolic Health. J of Obes. 2019, 8031705. DOI:10.1155/2019/8031705
59. Salvestrini V, Sell C, Lorenzini A. Obesity May Accelerate the Aging Process. Front. Endocrinol. 2019, DOI: 10.3389/fendo.2019.00266
60. Siparsky PN, Kirkendall DT, Garrett WE Jr. Muscle changes in aging: understanding sarcopenia. Sports Health. 2014, 6:1; 36-40. DOI:10.1177/1941738113502296
61. Colman RJ, Anderson RM. Nonhuman primate calorie restriction. Antioxid Redox Signal. 2011;14(2):229-239. DOI: 10.1089/ars.2010.3224
62. Feng Z, Lin M, Wu R. The Regulation of Aging and Longevity: A New and Complex Role of p53. Genes Cancer. 2011, 2:4; 443-52. DOI:10.1177/1947601911410223
63. Kaeberlein M, McVey M, Guarente L. The SIR2/3/4 complex and SIR2 alone promote longevity in Saccharomyces cerevisiae by two different mechanisms. Genes Dev. 1999, 13:19; 2570–80. DOI: 10.1101/gad.13.19.2570
64. Vinod N. Metabolic Disequilibrium and Aging: Modifying Favorably with Calorie Restriction and Calorie Restriction Mimetics. Gerontol & Geriatric stud. 2019, 4(5). GGS.000596.2019. DOI: 10.31031/GGS.2019.04.000596

65. Demine S, Renard P, Arnould T. Mitochondrial Uncoupling: A Key Controller of Biological Processes in Physiology and Diseases. Cells. 2019, 8:8; 795. DOI:10.3390/cells8080795

66. Murphy T, Dias GP, Thuret S. Effects of diet on brain plasticity in animal and human studies: mind the gap. Neural Plast. 2014, 563160. DOI:10.1155/2014/563160

67. Austad SN, Fischer KE. Sex Differences in Lifespan. Cell Metab. 2016, 23:6; 1022-33. DOI: 10.1016/j.cmet.2016.05.019

68. Liu, X., Tao, L., Cao, K. et al. Association of high-density lipoprotein with development of metabolic syndrome components: a five-year follow-up in adults. BMC Public Health, 2015, 15:412; DOI: 10.1186/s12889-015-1747-9

69. Moen OM. The case for cryonics. Journal of Medical Ethics, 2015, 41; 677-81. DOI: 10.1136/medethics-2015-102715

70. Vinod N. Future Projections and Fallouts of Exponential Longevity and Revival from Cryopreservation. Res Med Eng Sci. 6(4), RMES.000640.2018. DOI: 10.31031/RMES.2018.06.000640

71. Cerullo MA. The Ethics of Exponential Life Extension through Brain Preservation. Journal of Evolution and Technology, 2016, 26:1; 94-105

72. Eth D, Foust JC, Whale B. The Prospects of Whole Brain Emulation within the next Half- Century. Journal of Artificial General Intelligence, 2013, 4:3; DOI: 10.2478/jagi-2013-0008

73. Amunts K, Ebell C, Muller J, et al. The Human Brain Project: Creating a European Research Infrastructure to Decode the Human Brain. Neuron, 2016, 92:3, 574-81. DOI: 10.1016/j.neuron.2016.10.046

74. Morley JE. Tithonusism: Is it reversible? In - Endocrinology of Aging. (Eds.) Morley J.E., van den Berg L. Contemporary Endocrinology, 2000, vol 20, 11-21. Humana Press. ISBN: 978-1-61737-171-4. DOI:10.1007/978-1-59259-715-4_2

75. Gruenberg EM. The Failures of Success. The Milbank Memorial Fund Quarterly, 2005. 55:1, 1977, 3–24. DOI: 10.1111/j.1468-0009.2005.00400.x

76. Nikhra V. Exploring COVID-19: Perspectives and Patterns. Scholars' Press, June 2020, ISBN-13: 978-613-8-93051-8, ISBN-10: 6138930517, www.scholars-press.com

77. Al-Rawi Y. Editorial - When Tithonus met corona: the COVID-19 pandemic and acute illness in the elderly. BMJ Supportive & Palliative Care Published Online, 24 June 2020. DOI: 10.1136/bmjspcare-2020-002424

78. Shrivastava SR, Shrivastava PS, Ramasamy J. Health-care of Elderly: Determinants, Needs and Services. Int J Prev Med. 2013, 4:10; 1224-25.

79. Halaweh H, Dahlin-Ivanoff S, Svantesson U, et al. Perspectives of Older Adults on Aging Well: A Focus Group Study. Journal of Aging Research 2018, Article ID 9858252, 9 pages, DOI: 10.1155/2018/9858252

80. Vance DE, Kaur J, Fazeli PL, et al. Neuroplasticity and successful cognitive aging: a brief overview for nursing. J Neurosci Nurs. 2012, 44:4; 218-227. DOI: 10.1097/JNN.0b013e3182527571

81. Basso JC, Suzuki WA. The Effects of Acute Exercise on Mood, Cognition, Neurophysiology, and Neurochemical Pathways: A Review. Brain Plast. 2017, 2:2; 127-152. DOI:10.3233/BPL-160040

82. Booth FW, Roberts CK, Laye MJ. Lack of exercise is a major cause of chronic diseases. Comprehensive Physiology 2012, 2:2; 1143-1211. DOI:10.1002/cphy.c110025

83. Institute of Medicine (US) Subcommittee on Military Weight Management. Weight Management: State of the Science and Opportunities for Military Programs. Washington, DC: National Academies Press, US, 2004. 4, Weight-Loss and Maintenance Strategies. https://www.ncbi.nlm.nih.gov/books/NBK221839/

84. Powers SK, Smuder AJ, Kavazis AN, et al. Mechanisms of exercise-induced cardioprotection. Physiology (Bethesda), 2014, 29:1; 27-38. DOI:10.1152/physiol.00030.2013

85. Stover PJ. Vitamin B12 and older adults. Curr Opin Clin Nutr Metab Care. 2010, 13:1; 24-27. DOI: 10.1097/MCO.0b013e328333d157

86. Sgarbieri VC, Pacheco MTB. Healthy human aging: intrinsic and environmental factors. Braz. J. Food Technol. 2017, Vol 20. DOI: 10.1590/1981-6723.00717

87. Lobo V, Patil A, Phatak A, et al. Free radicals, antioxidants and functional foods: Impact on human health. Pharmacogn Rev. 2010, 4:8; 118-126. DOI:10.4103/0973-7847.70902

88. Scalbert A, Andres-Lacueva C, Arita M, et al. Databases on food phytochemicals and their health-promoting effects. J Agric Food Chem. 2011, 59:9; 4331-48. DOI:10.1021/jf200591d

89. Sui Z, Wong WK, Louie JCY, et al. Discretionary food and beverage consumption and its association with demographic characteristics, weight status, and fruit and vegetable intakes in Australian adults. Public Health Nutrition 2017, 20:2, 274-81. DOI:10.1017/S1368980016002305

90. Forni C, Facchiano F, Bartoli M, et al. Beneficial Role of Phytochemicals on Oxidative Stress and Age-Related Diseases. Biomed Res Int. 2019, 8748253. DOI:10.1155/2019/8748253

91. Snopek L, Mlcek J, Sochorova L, et al. Contribution of Red Wine Consumption to Human Health Protection. Molecules. 2018, 23:7; 1684. DOI:10.3390/molecules23071684

92. Guddeti RR, Dang G, Williams MA, et al. Role of Yoga in Cardiac Disease and Rehabilitation. Journal of Cardiopulmonary Rehabilitation and Prevention, 2019, 39:3; 146-152. DOI: 10.1097/HCR.0000000000000372

93. Jahnke R, Larkey L, Rogers C, et al. A comprehensive review of health benefits of qigong and tai chi. Am J Health Promot 2010, 24:6; e1-e25. DOI: 10.4278/ajhp.081013-LIT-248.

94. Garcia JM, Merriam GR, Kargi AY. Growth Hormone in Aging. [Updated 2019]. In: Feingold KR, Anawalt B, Boyce A, et al., editors. Endotext. South Dartmouth (MA): MDText.com, Inc.; 2000-. https://www.ncbi.nlm.nih.gov/books/NBK279163/

95. Kaufman JM, Vermeulen A. The decline of androgen levels in elderly men and its clinical and therapeutic implications. Endocr Rev. 2005, 26:6; 833-76. DOI:10.1210/er.2004-0013.

96. Walther A, Seuffert J. Testosterone and Dehydroepiandrosterone Treatment in Ageing Men: Are We All Set? World J Mens Health. 2020, 38:2; 178-190. DOI: 10.5534/wjmh.190006

97. Ahern T, Wu FCW. New horizons in testosterone and the ageing male. Age and Ageing, 2015, 44:2; 188–95. DOI: 10.1093/ageing/afv007

98. Li Y, Li S, Zhou Y, et al. Melatonin for the prevention and treatment of cancer. Oncotarget. 2017, 8:24, 39896-39921. DOI: 10.18632/oncotarget.16379

99. Orallo F. Comparative studies of the antioxidant effects of cis- and trans-resveratrol. Curr Med Chem. 2006, 13:1; 87-98.

100. Kfoury C. Therapeutic cloning: promises and issues. Mcgill J Med. 2007, 10:2; 112-120.

101. Rowan S, Bejarano E, Taylor A. Mechanistic targeting of advanced glycation end-products in age-related diseases. Biochimica et Biophysica Acta (BBA) - Molecular Basis of Disease. 2018, 1864:12; 3631-43. DOI: 10.1016/j.bbadis.2018.08.036

102. Samper E, Flores JM, Blasco MA. Restoration of telomerase activity rescues chromosomal instability and premature aging in Terc-/- mice with short telomeres. EMBO Rep. 2001, 2:9; 800-807. DOI:10.1093/embo-reports/kve174

103. Nazari-Shafti TZ, Cooke JP. Telomerase Therapy to Reverse Cardiovascular Senescence. Methodist Debakey Cardiovasc J. 2015, 11:3; 172-175. DOI:10.14797/mdcj-11-3-172

<u>COMMUNICATION TO THE AUTHOR</u>

*Please communicate your
opinion, feedback, and suggestions
to the author at*

drvinodnikhra@gmail.com

Facebook: drvinodnikhra

Instagram: vnikhra

Twitter: Vnikhra

www.vinodnikhra.com